T0373674

LEADERSHIP LESSONS FROM A GLOBAL HEALTH CRISIS

This book explores the key learning concepts for global leadership in the face of modern international health crises and argues the need for fundamental reform to governance paradigms, within the global security sphere and policymaking circles. Beginning with an analysis of the worldwide response to the COVID-19 pandemic, the book provides insights from evolution, history, and human behaviour to explain how our current leadership paradigms have contributed to today's global health challenges and draws lessons for the much larger crisis of climate change with the threat of massive biodiversity collapse. The second part of the book outlines tangible solutions to transform leadership and policy to enhance global security for both people and the planet, with the aim of averting future pandemics and our planetary emergency.

This book:

Will be among the first published works to examine the international response to the COVID-19 pandemic, and draws valuable lessons for our climate crisis.

Directly addresses the nexus between scientific advice and policymaking, highlighting recommendations for future leaders.

Provides a bridge between public health, the environment, and leadership.

This book will prove an insightful resource for current and future world leaders, politicians, and policymakers, as well as environmental and public health professional bodies, think tanks, and institutions shaping the next generation of leadership.

Dr. Jo Nurse is a strategic advisor to the InterAction Council, a group of 40 former international leaders and Heads of Government currently chaired by HE Bertie Ahern and HE President Obasanjo, advancing collaborative initiatives to enhance governance for global security for people and the planet. Prior to this, Jo was Head of Health and Education for the Commonwealth, providing leadership to ministers across 53 countries, and strengthening systems and capacity for the education and health sectors to enable sustainable development. Earlier in her career, Jo was the UK government's national lead for Public Mental Health and Wellbeing developing multi-sector policies to promote wider well-being including the prevention of violence. From 2010, Jo worked for the World Health Organization, developing capacity for climate change assessments and strategies, led the implementation of the WHO European Action Plan for Public Health, and applied this experience as a key architect of the World Federation of Public Health Associations 'Global Charter for the Public's Health'. Jo is currently advancing these initiatives as Director for the Platform for Planet, Place and People, a hub of the Commonwealth Centre for Digital Health. Having held a number of honorary professorships, Jo was recently made a fellow of the World Academy of Art and Science and chairs a group on Existential Threats to Humanity.

Routledge Focus on Environmental Health
Series Editor: Stephen Battersby, MBE PhD, FCIEH, FRSPH

Housing, Health and Well-Being
Stephen Battersby, Véronique Ezratty and David Ormandy

Selective Licensing
The Basis for a Collaborative Approach to Addressing Health Inequalities
Paul Oatt

Assessing Public Health Needs in a Lower Middle Income Country
Sarah Ruel-Bergeron, Jimi Patel, Riksum Kazi and Charlotte Burch

Fire Safety in Residential Property
A Practical Approach for Environmental Health
Richard Lord

COVID-19: The Global Environmental Health Experience
Chris Day

Regulating the Privately Rented Housing Sector
Evidence into Practice
Edited by Jill Stewart and Russell Moffatt

Dampness in Dwellings
Causes and Effects
David Ormandy, Véronique Ezratty and Stephen Battersby

Tackling Environmental Health Inequalities in a South African City?
Rediscovering Regulation, Local Government and its Environmental Health
Practitioners
Rob Couch

Leadership Lessons from a Global Health Crisis

From the Pandemic to the Climate Emergency

Dr. Jo Nurse

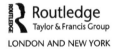

Routledge
Taylor & Francis Group

LONDON AND NEW YORK

First published 2023
by Routledge
4 Park Square, Milton Park, Abingdon, Oxon OX14 4RN

and by Routledge
605 Third Avenue, New York, NY 10158

Routledge is an imprint of the Taylor & Francis Group, an informa business

British Library Cataloguing-in-Publication Data
A catalogue record for this book is available from the British Library

ISBN: 978-1-032-01003-8 (hbk)
ISBN: 978-1-032-01939-0 (pbk)
ISBN: 978-1-003-18108-8 (ebk)

DOI: 10.1201/9781003181088

Typeset in Times New Roman
by codeMantra

Contents

Figures

Series Preface

This is the thirteenth publication in the series, with more in the pipeline. This edition, like the previous edition, reflects our desire to highlight environmental health work and issues around the world. There are lessons that environmental health practitioners (EHP) and policymakers can learn from colleagues working in different settings and in the variety of social, political, and legal structures. It has also been fundamental to environmental health that prevention is better than cure, and as this work shows, it is more cost-effective if it is embedded into other sectors, with a One Health approach covering resilience, security, emergencies, animals, and the environment. Fundamentally, the aim must be to protect public health that is prevention of ill-health and unintentional injuries. As this edition shows, this requires leadership, and sadly the COVID-19 pandemic and the climate crisis show this has not always been there. So this is perhaps a challenge for EHPs.

This edition further illustrates the flexibility offered by the series, but the aim remains as ever; to explore environmental health topics traditional or new and raise sometimes contentious issues in more detail than might be found in the usual environmental health texts. It is a means whereby environmental health issues can be discussed with a wider audience in mind. The author has worked at the World Health Organization and the Commonwealth Secretariat as well and is an advisor to the InterAction Council – a group of 40 former Heads of Government with an emphasis on global security. This shows the range of potential authors who could contribute to the series.

This series is an important part of the professional landscape. Environmental and public health practitioners bring their expertise to a range of situations and are deployed differently but not always to the best effect. All too often politicians both at the national and local levels are complacent, are unaware of what is environmental health, and what practitioners do or how they work. It is common that practitioners have a 'low profile' or are taken for granted. It is hoped that this series will be used as a means of highlighting environmental and public health issues and the work of practitioners.

We also want to encourage colleagues, particularly those who might not have had work published previously, to submit proposals as we hope to be responsive to the needs of environmental and public health practitioners. I am particularly keen that this series is seen as an opportunity for first-time authors and as ever would urge students (whether at first- or second-degree level) to consider this an avenue for publishing findings from their research. Why for example should the hard work that has gone into a dissertation or thesis lie unread on a library shelf? We can provide advice on turning a thesis into a book. Equally, this series can be a way of extending a presentation, paper, or training materials, so that these can reach a wider audience.

The series provides a route for practitioners to improve the profile of the profession either directly or indirectly by using the works to advocate on policy, as well as to provide a source of information. It has the advantage of having a relatively quick turnaround from submission of the manuscript to publication and can be more up to date and immediate than a standard text-book or reference work.

It remains a concern that EHPs wherever employed have perhaps not been good at telling others about their work. To be considered a genuine profession and to develop professionally EHPs on the front line need to 'get published', writing up their work of protecting public health. This is a route for analysing actions and reporting on what worked in practice, what was successful what wasn't and why. This can provide useful insights for others working in the field and also highlight policy issues of relevance to environmental health.

Contributing to this series should not be seen merely as an exercise in gathering Continual Professional Development (CPD) hours but as a useful method of reflection and aid to career development, something that anyone who considers themselves a professional should do. I am pleased to be working with Routledge to provide this opportunity for practitioners.

As has been made clear, and this edition highlights, it is not intended that this series takes a wholly 'technical' approach but provides an opportunity to consider areas of policy and practice in a different way, for example, looking at the social and political aspects of environmental health in addition to a more discursive approach on specialist areas.

Our hope remains that this is a dynamic series, providing a forum for new ideas and debate on environmental health topics. If readers have any ideas for titles in the series, please do not be afraid to submit them to me as series editor via the e-mail addresses below.

'Environmental health' can be taken to mean different things in different countries around the world and so we welcome suggestions from a range of professionals doing 'environmental health' work or policy development. EHPs may be a key part of the public health workforce wherever they practise, but there are also many other practitioners working to safeguard public and environmental health. It is hoped that this series will enable a wider range of practitioners and others with a professional interest to access information and also to write about issues relevant to them.

Forthcoming monographs will cover such topics as air pollution and sewage pollution. We are in contact with colleagues around the world encouraging them to submit proposals. That does not mean we have no need of further suggestions, quite the contrary, so I hope readers with ideas for a monograph will get in touch via Ed.Needle@tandf.co.uk

Stephen Battersby MBE PhD, FCIEH, FRSPH

Series Editor

Foreword

Collectively, we failed to prevent the catastrophic impacts of the COVID-19 pandemic. We cannot afford to fail again. Together, we must ensure that we succeed with tackling our planetary emergency.

The COVID-19 pandemic revealed weaknesses in how we deal with threats to human life, health, and civilisation. Although some countries managed to contain the virus, our collective emergency plans and systems suffered many failings. Despite a variety of efforts, more than three years on, we are still vulnerable to the impacts of another pandemic.

It is evident that our current systems are failing to protect us from increasingly complex and interconnected challenges to our human security. Human life and survival are entirely reliant on having a healthy planet to live upon. This requires a coordinated multilateral governance system to ensure global security for people and the planet.

Within our reach, we have the solutions to create a safer world. We know how to strengthen and ensure cost-effective public and environmental health services at community and national levels. The key to successful prevention includes being prepared for risks, monitoring for early detection, and ensuring swift and coordinated responses. Digital and innovative solutions are already available that can offer these functions as a global good.

Leaders must be equipped to deal with emergencies and know how to react to threats to our survival. To be successful, we must create a fail-safe international infrastructure that coordinates a strategic response as part of our global security system.

This book builds upon a series of High-Level Expert Meetings convened by the InterAction Council on global health threats – ranging from the Ebola crisis to the planetary emergency and the pandemic. The InterAction Council is a group of roughly 40 former world leaders who are committed to creating a safer and more sustainable world together.

The first part of the book analyses how and why we failed in our collective response to the pandemic and includes valuable insights into human nature and emotional reactions to existential threats. Future risks from pandemics, as well as global threats to our health, life, and existence are also outlined.

The second part of the book presents solutions for preventing future pandemics with lessons for responding effectively to our planetary emergency. These include the application of digital technology to create modern one-planet health systems that build upon effective public and environmental health operations.

Lastly, the role of education and training of future leaders to deal with complex threats is outlined, to be supported by leadership and governance systems that enhance human security.

I wholeheartedly welcome this book, written by Dr. Joanna Nurse, an advisor to the InterAction Council, which provides timely and valuable lessons for how, together, we can create a safer and healthier world, where everyone can flourish.

Thomas S Axworthy
Secretary-General, InterAction Council

Preface

The era of COVID-19 pandemic has created a significant shift in political, economic, and social dynamics around the world, presenting humanity with the opportunity for profound learning in its response to our planetary crisis. A key lesson that has emerged is that when faced with an emergency, human nature does not always respond in beneficial ways. As these can be seen as repeating patterns in multiple settings, the first part of this book explores how and why we respond to such threats, in order to gain insight to ensure that our leaders are more resilient in responding to emergencies in the future. The other significant reflection is that we cannot afford to rely upon individual leaders to always respond appropriately to unexpected and unknown emergencies. We need to ensure that we invest in the infrastructure required to avert future disasters.

As climate change accelerates relentlessly, we need to ensure that we do not fail in our collective endeavours to create a safe and sustainable world for all. To achieve this, we need to redesign and strengthen our emergency governance mechanisms, in order to avert global catastrophe. Therefore, the second part of this book draws upon the learning from the pandemic and provides an outline of how to strengthen skills for our emergency governance and leadership systems. Strengthening public health and environmental health operations and modernising the workforce to create a multi-sector 'One-Planet Health System' will be key to addressing threats to our health and life. Applying digital solutions has the potential to transform our human security as a global good. The book concludes with a blueprint for enhancing Global Security for Planet and People to provide the international infrastructure required to secure our collective futures from pandemics and our planetary emergency.

Dr Jo Nurse, Strategic Advisor, The InterAction Council
BMed, MSc, MPH, PhD, MRCGP, FFPH, FWAAS.

'In our interconnected world, multilateralism and co-ordination are essential to successfully containing and combating virus outbreaks'.

Olusegun Obasanjo, former President of Nigeria: Co-chair of the InterAction Council.

'Global health security affects us all. The Covid-19 pandemic is providing us with countless learning opportunities. We all hope to emerge stronger, but we have an opportunity to also emerge better. Let us reflect on not only the lessons of this time of crisis but also on the years prior. When we rebuild, let's do it right. Our goal must be to build a healthier planet'.

Bertie Ahern, former Prime Minister of Ireland: Co-chair of the InterAction Council.

https://www.interactioncouncil.org/media-centre/council-former-world-leaders-urges-urgent-global-co-operation-combat-covid-19-and-plan

Acknowledgements

For all their patience, support, and inspiration, I would especially like to thank my partner Helen and close family members including Jules and Richard. The learning that I have shared in this book comes from the exceptionally valuable insights gained from advising the InterAction Council. In particular, I would like to express my appreciation to all the wise leaders of the InterAction Council, and the encouragement to write this book by their SG, Thomas Axworthy, and Tanya Guy. A special note of thanks goes to Nicholas Fogg for his dedicated editing, as well as the balanced reflections from Moneef Zou'bi.

This book builds upon a series of the InterAction Council High-Level Expert Group meetings, including their summary reports and recommendations. I wish to thank the many professional partners and experts who have contributed to these meetings that have informed reports and shaped this book. In particular, I express my gratitude to the environmental health leaders Stephen Battersby and Peter Archer for all their longstanding commitment and who made this book possible. Thanks is given to all the formal professional feedback and endorsements for the InterAction Council reports that this book builds upon, with a special acknowledgement for in-depth discussions into the contents of this book from Fiona Adshead and Karen Lock. My continued gratitude goes to Vajira Dissanayake and all the Commonwealth Digital Health Fellows who serve the world in the creation of digital health solutions as a common good. My deep respect is especially conveyed to Josephine Ojiambo and Winnie Kiap for their valuable insights into political power and human nature.

The lives of all those who died as a consequence of the COVID-19 pandemic, along with the exceptional dedication and endurance of frontline workers and professionals responding to the pandemic, are gratefully acknowledged. This book has been written to ensure that we learn from this catastrophe to create a safer world together.

Last but by no means least, I wish to dedicate this book to two people who are no longer with us: John Wyn Owen, for his wise and humble leadership as a mentor and an advisor to the InterAction Council, and to my Mother who embraced everyone with her heart.

1 Learning from the Pandemic – A Crisis of Leadership

The Pandemic – A Failure of Leadership?

Collectively, we have failed in our response to avert untold deaths, disabilities, and devastations from the COVID-19 pandemic. Since the pandemic was officially declared by the World Health Organization (WHO) in 2020, it appears that we sleep-walked into an avoidable global catastrophe. We had many warnings, and many opportunities to have potentially averted this tragedy, so why did we not intervene earlier to prevent it, act swiftly to eliminate its spread, or apply existing knowledge and public health measures to contain this unfolding disaster? Maybe we were falsely reassured by our relative success in preventing the SARS outbreak, or the Ebola epidemic, both significantly more fatal viruses, from spreading into pandemics, and were thus lulled into a sense that we could easily manage what seemed to be the relatively mild coronavirus, COVID-19.

Ultimately though, we cannot claim that we did not know about the risks of a pandemic – scientists had alerted governments that another significant pandemic could occur at any point. Consequently, many governments and the World Economic Forum had placed the risk of a pandemic high upon their risk registers. The 2019 Global Preparedness Monitoring Board report 'A World at Risk' (GPMB, 2019) warned that there was 'a very real threat of a rapidly spreading pandemic due to a lethal respiratory pathogen'. It emphasised the importance of the role of Heads of Government in ensuring financial risk planning for adequate investment to strengthen preparedness and coordinated systems, both nationally and internationally. The Commission for a Global Health Risk Framework for the Future (NAM, 2016) recommended an annual global investment of US$ 4.5 billion for pandemic preparedness, including public health preventative measures and research. Such sums pall in comparison to the Economist's estimate that global GDP had shrunk between 4.3% and 6.6% in 2020, and as of March 2021, the Economist estimated the economic cost of the COVID-19 pandemic at $10 trillion (Economist, 2021). Whilst, the World Bank (2022) issued a warning that the global economy might be on the brink of 'Stagflation', consisting of the brutal combination

DOI: 10.1201/9781003181088-1

of low economic growth and high inflation, which was precipitated by the pandemic and the Russian invasion of Ukraine.

This new era of pandemics and planetary emergencies is fundamentally challenging the ability of existing governance and leadership systems to respond to increasingly complex global threats. It has revealed our human fragility and highlighted how interconnected all our lives are across the world. Thus, there is an urgent need to review such lessons and apply learning to transform governance mechanisms that ensure the prevention of a reoccurrence of a pandemic on this scale. As emphasised by the InterAction Council of former Heads of State and Government in its 'Dublin Charter for One Health', we need to enhance links between the Health of the Planet and the Health of People (IAC, 2017). Ultimately, though due to the gravity of the consequences to human civilisation, we cannot afford to fail in our response to this planetary emergency. The devastation that resulted from the Second World War led to the establishment of the United Nations and the transformation of health and education systems in many parts of the world. In a similar way, the pandemic represents a key opportunity to ensure that we succeed in our collective endeavours to avert a further catastrophe from unfolding.

Pandemic Imperialism – A Threat to Global Security

The COVID-19 pandemic has been brutal and far reaching in its impacts – with over 6 million deaths recorded directly from COVID-19 by the WHO by the middle of 2022, with an estimated 15 million excess deaths during 2020–2021 (WHO, 2022). In contrast, the Institute for Health Metrics and Evaluation has estimated over 18 million excess deaths related directly and indirectly to COVID-19 (Wang et al, 2022). Moreover, the pandemic has acted as a significant social disruptor, creating chaos and uncertainty with last-minute lockdowns that have resulted in mass unemployment, increased stress levels, and domestic abuse, as well as a loss of educational and future opportunities for young people. The impacts have disproportionately affected disadvantaged people and reinforced long-standing inequalities, including ageism, racism, and increased discrimination against people with disabilities. At the global level, long-standing injustices and inequities have been played out with regard to unequal access to vaccines. The pandemic has also resulted in significant political disruption, with public outrage and riots, and elections being lost and won based upon the apparent ability of political leaders to limit and respond to the impacts of COVID-19. In turn, it has threatened wider global security and stability and the capacity to deliver on Sustainable Development Goals and may continue to do so for many years.

The influence of the power dynamics of a handful of higher-income countries continues to have a disproportionate influence in shaping global health policies and outcomes. A vivid illustration of such 'Pandemic Imperialism' is demonstrated in the unequal distribution of COVID-19 vaccines. In June

2022, the WHO reported that only 58 of its 194 member states had achieved 70% vaccination coverage, but virtually all were high-income countries (WHO, 2022). In contrast, nearly one billion people in lower-income countries were still unvaccinated. The reasons for this level of vaccine inequality are multiple – including vaccine hoarding by wealthy countries, the predominance of vaccine research, and suppliers and pharmaceutical companies being based within high-income countries, which have held onto knowledge, finances, and vaccines for their own benefit. It took over two years from the start of the pandemic for the World Trade Organization to reach an agreement for a patent waiver for COVID-19 vaccines allowing all countries to produce and export vaccines – the agreement, however, excluded COVID-19 diagnostics and therapeutics. In a world where people matter more than wealth, collaborative vaccine development and distribution could have occurred as a common good.

Moreover, countries that allowed COVID-19 to spread at high levels across their communities have contributed to the development of new variants and continued worldwide waves of the pandemic. With failed commitments to protect the world through vaccination, the default national response of several G7 and G20 countries shifted the global narrative towards allowing COVID-19 to become endemic ('Herd Immunity'). The predominance of this narrative undermined other countries' efforts to protect their populations with what had been initially successful elimination and exit strategies. This can be seen as a form of 'Pandemic Imperialism' – whereby countries that have pursued national policies without due consideration for their impact upon the rest of the world have caused untold preventable deaths and widening social and economic inequalities. Some advocates have expressed these situations as a crime against humanity – with a case already made for over 600,000 deaths of Brazilians including a disproportionate number of indigenous citizens (Dyer, 2021). The report recommended that charges are filed against President Bolsonaro, including the propagation of pathogenic germs and crimes against humanity; these charges have since been submitted to the International Criminal Court (ABJD, 2021).

There have, however, been significant paradoxes, with some countries with High- and Middle-Income Gross National Incomes having been devastated by the COVID-19 pandemic, when they appeared to have been prepared with some of the strongest public health systems in the world. This tended to occur in countries in which the political stance ranged from playing down to even denying the pandemic. In other countries, the scientific community voiced fatalistic scenarios that led to the single perspective that the only solution was the adoption of 'herd immunity' – in essence allowing the virus to become endemic in order to build a national pool of resistance. Unfortunately, the narrative of learning to live with COVID and allowing it to become endemic appears to have been the highest-risk approach as the more the virus has been allowed to spread, the greater the chance of new variants developing

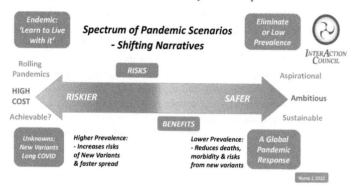

Figure 1.1 Pandemic Imperialist Narratives Create a Shift to an Endemic State

with further pandemic waves. Modelling predicts that this process could take at least ten years for a more stable endemic state to be achieved. This, however, assumes that no new variants will occur. Moreover, from a viral immunological perspective, future COVID mutations will not necessarily become milder and could as well become more harmful (IAC, 2022). Figure 1.1 illustrates how the predominance of pandemic narratives has led to the pandemic becoming endemic.

A Scientific Start to the COVID-19 Pandemic

The first indications of a new virus emerging were picked up at the end of December 2019 by the WHO Country Office in China, which had identified media reports from the city of Wuhan of a cluster of cases of a viral pneumonia. On December 31, the Country Office informed the International Health Regulations (IHR) focal point for the WHO Western Pacific Regional Office of this. The next day, the WHO Incident Management Support Team met to coordinate responses and offer support to China. Soon after, the Global Outbreak Alert and Response Network (GOARN) informed public health agencies, laboratories, and international organisations of the impending crisis. On January 5, the WHO issued its first Disease Outbreak News Report on the new viral pneumonia to the global media and on its public website. On January 9, the Chinese authorities identified the cause of the outbreak as a novel coronavirus. In response, on January 10, the WHO convened its Strategic and Technical Advisory Group on Infectious Hazards as well as its Research and Development Advisory and Coordination Groups.

On January 13, the first case of the disease outside of China was reported in Thailand. On January 15, the Japanese Health Ministry reported that a man in Kanagawa province had tested positive for the virus. He had recently visited Wuhan. The announcement of the first reported case in the USA on

January 21 coincided with an announcement by the WHO that there was evidence of human-to-human transmission. On January 22 and 23, Dr. Tedros Adhanom Ghebreyesus, Director-General of the WHO, convened an International Health Regulations Emergency Committee (IHR EC) of 15 independent experts, largely consisting of Heads of Infectious Disease Institutes and academics from around the world. They were charged with advising the Director-General on whether the outbreak constituted a 'Public Health Emergency of International Concern' (PHEIC). As they considered that there was insufficient information and no intermediate level of warning existed, the committee decided not to issue a PHEIC. On January 27 and 28, Dr. Tedros Adhanom Ghebreyesus visited China as Director-General of the WHO to learn more about the outbreak. On his return, he reconvened the IHR EC. With 98 reported cases in 18 countries outside of China, it was decided that the outbreak did now indeed constitute a 'PHEIC'. The Director-General issued a statement to that effect on January 30th, 2020.

During February 2020, the WHO updated and finalised its operational guidance including its Strategic Preparedness and Response Plan and the Secretary-General of the United Nations activated its crisis management policy. Following the deployment of a further mission to China, on February 11 and 12, the WHO convened a Global Research and Innovation Forum of over 300 experts and funders to accelerate the finance necessary to understand the nature of the virus and identify potential vaccines and treatments. This was followed by the publication of a Global Research Roadmap on March 6. The Director-General continued to raise awareness and mobilise resources through regular press releases, weekly Member State meetings, and a presentation at the Munich Security Conference, where he expressed concern at the lack of global urgency and funding. Due to the perceived confusion of the term 'Public Health Emergency of International Concern' (PHEIC) originally announced on January 30, combined with continued inaction and the alarming rate of the spread of the contagion, on March 11th, the WHO declared that COVID-19 could be characterised as a 'Pandemic'. This announcement, together with media coverage of Italy's health systems becoming overwhelmed by the spread of the virus, soon led to the declaration of national emergencies and lockdowns across much of Europe and North America.

Such was the spread of the new virus that, within 100 days of its first reportage, there were over 1 million cases detected worldwide, a clear indication of the power of globalisation. Within the first year of the announcement of the pandemic, over 2.5 million deaths were reported. In this context, the global and national responses to the pandemic can be seen as too late, too slow, and too inadequate to have prevented millions of excess deaths and disabilities, as well as the unfolding of longer-term social-economic damage. During the first months of 2020, there were a number of potentially missed opportunities that could have prevented the pandemic from escalating and contained the widespread harm it caused or have sought a strategy of elimination.

In retrospect, the predominance of a science-led response to the pandemic resulted in the use of overly technical language which slowed the perception of risk. This was due to the group of experts advising on whether to declare a 'PHEIC' largely coming from medical and research backgrounds. This was further reinforced by the predominance of scientific experts leading the initial response. Although the use of such experts was important in dealing with a health emergency and fortunately resulted in the development of effective vaccines, it limited the public health measures and emergency levers that they could have utilised. This can be seen by the initial response in February 2000 that convened a large research meeting to study the virus, as opposed to convening Health Ministers, professional leaders, and Heads of National Institutes of Public Health to coordinate a global emergency response at speed.

Significantly, relying predominately upon those with a research background led to a research response, which requires considerable time to test hypotheses and develop solutions that are not always applicable to scaling up through policy or existing operational systems. With COVID-19, it was fortuitous that a vaccine was developed through immense research and pharmaceutical funding. Yet vaccines may not always be possible for future pandemics, for example, there is still no effective vaccine for HIV. A wider skills-mix of risk analysts, public health, and emergency professionals together with clearer communications targeted at political leaders and decision-makers during the early stages of the pandemic could have prevented a global emergency from unfolding on such a scale. As was demonstrated with other emerging pandemics such as SARS and MERS, time is of the essence, with an initial emphasis upon prevention and containment to stop the pandemic from spreading which allows the possibility of adopting an elimination strategy.

The Absence of Architecture for Global Health Security

In some respects, the COVID-19 epidemic can be seen as a fortunate test run, as it highlighted the many weaknesses in our emergency systems, as a relatively mild infection with a low fatality rate. In the future, with the emergence of new variants, we may not be so lucky – especially if a new virus has a higher fatality rate and spreads more easily. In order to succeed in preventing future pandemics and in applying learning to avert our planetary emergency, we need to draw key lessons from this pandemic. One of the main functions of government is to ensure the security of its population, and a key focus of this book is the role of leaders and leadership systems in responding to emergencies. Moreover, stronger links are needed between the role that health plays in contributing to global security and the application and modernisation of existing global security measures to prevent and respond to health threats. The next section outlines the international response and illustrates the incredible effort made by the WHO to garner a global response, but the fact that it needed to do so in the midst of a pandemic highlights the absence of a pre-existent infrastructure that could have created a rapid global strategic response.

During 2020, the WHO continued to provide regular communications and guidance documents, as well as to advocate for increased funding and joint efforts with United Nations' partners and within a variety of international forums. In March 2020, the Director-General spoke at the G20 Extraordinary Summit on COVID-19, which ended with a statement of solidarity to work with the WHO to strengthen health systems globally and finance the response to the pandemic. On April 20, 2020, the UN General Assembly adopted a resolution calling for 'International cooperation to ensure global access to medicines, vaccines and medical equipment to face COVID-19'. That acknowledged the crucial role of the WHO in leading the response, followed shortly afterwards by the establishment of the COVID-19 Tools Accelerator, which later in the year advanced vaccine development, and equity of access through the COVAX initiative.

The WHO is the organisation mandated by the United Nations as its leader on health, with the role of advocating for and providing health information, standards and technical expertise, building capacity, and developing global strategies and plans, including those for health emergencies. In May 2020, Health Ministers met virtually at the annual World Health Assembly, with 14 heads of state participating: a call was made to intensify efforts to control the pandemic, whilst the Director-General also instigated an independent review of the pandemic (IPPPR, 2021). Since then, the WHO has maintained its efforts to advocate for vaccine equity, mobilise resources, provide pandemic information, guidance and standards, including joint United Nations initiatives, and enhance capacity within individual countries. During September 2020, at the UN General Assembly, the WHO called for world leaders to support access to the COVID-19 Tools Accelerator initiatives and convened sessions on mitigating the impact of COVID-19, stopping the spread of misinformation and improving emergency preparedness. Whilst the United Nations Security Council has convened a number of sessions on the issue, the main resolution and focus have been on a cessation of international hostilities in order to prioritise the combating of the pandemic.

In December 2020, almost a year after the initial emergence of the new coronavirus, the United Nations hosted a summit on COVID-19, which mainly emphasised multilateral action to raise funds towards the COVID-19 Tools Accelerator initiatives, including vaccine equity. However, attendance was often delegated to Health Ministers, and there was an overreliance on contributions by scientists and health experts, which maintained the status quo and only provided a limited political perspective on the pandemic. In marked contrast, the United Nations Security Council Summit on Post-COVID-19 Global Governance, chaired by the President of Niger in September 2020, highlighted the structural limitations of the current multilateral security system in dealing with global challenges such as pandemics and climate change, and called for global governance reform to enhance the convergence of sustainable peace and security. This meeting provided valuable reflections that can be applied to shape the future global security architecture which will be explored later in this book.

In retrospect, from the perspective of many politicians and policymakers, the pandemic seemed to emerge with little warning and escalated and overwhelmed countries at a speed to which governments struggled to respond. Not surprisingly, this in turn led to leaders focusing on the internal crisis, at times emphasising a nationalistic response, leaving little room to engage with, and provide strategic direction to external and multilateral global responses. At global level, it can be seen that political leaders delegated responsibility to the WHO as the designated lead agency, and the WHO did all that it could with such levers that were available to it. In contrast, at the national levels, an emergency situation response on this scale and impact is usually led and coordinated by the Head of Government, with the support of a high-level ministerial committee supported by a secretariat of policy officials, as this provides the level of leadership needed to garner the resources and coordinate the multi-sector responses that are required.

At a global level, placing the WHO as lead agency to respond to such a complex multi-sector emergency can be seen to have limited the multilateral response required due to the relative power that a health agency is perceived to have in comparison to that of a world leader or head of government. This may well have contributed to the relatively siloed health sector response to the pandemic, with its strong focus on health research and technical solutions, as these reflected the main levers open to the WHO. Additionally, this was likely to have been further reinforced by the 'group thinking' that occurred within a relatively narrow range of sectional expertise. The expert and technical language utilised to describe the severity of the situation appears to have further contributed to the relatively slow engagement by political leaders and policymakers in taking emergency action.

We can only reflect upon how this pandemic might have followed a very different pathway, had a global security mechanism already existed that mirrored that of many emergency systems that occur at a national level. Such a system could have possessed the governance infrastructure necessary to garner the political leadership and resources required for a swift, strategic, coordinated, multilateral, and multi-sector response to the emerging pandemic. Moving forward, a considered reform of the infrastructure of global security governance would be instrumental in averting future global emergencies such as pandemics and other potential health threats including those related to climate and biodiversity crises.

Rights versus Responsibilities and the Rise of Nationalist Responses

Early in 2020, as the emergence of this new coronavirus became evident, many political responses at the national level appeared slow and limited in scale, despite repeated warnings by the WHO of the perils of inaction. Initial responses ranged from denial and ignoring the outbreak, to a sense of what was occurring in China, 'could not possibly happen to us', to one of overconfidence in the preparedness of existing plans and systems. Later in February and March 2020, images of the health system in Italy rapidly becoming overwhelmed, led to a range of responses, including shock with initial inertia, to what appeared to be a growing sense of panic, with rapid changes in policy decisions, and then to a fluctuating attitude of bravado and overoptimism. In retrospect, these multiple responses reflect patterns of human behaviour that can occur in a crisis situation and will be explored further in later chapters.

These initial natural human responses to a crisis often resulted in an unfortunate pattern of unfolding chaos, which became further aggravated by the multiple uncertainties created by this unknown new virus. Countries that were unable to gather themselves together swiftly after the initial shock and establish a comprehensive emergency response with an adaptable strategic plan and coordinated delivery systems, appeared to be thrown into fluctuating cycles of panic. This was seen in the form of delayed and at times reversed decision-making, often focusing on single solutions, without apparent connection to existing policy or delivery systems. This approach resulted in fragmented and siloed responses without any clear coherence or coordination. An additional compounding factor was the pattern of increasingly insular leadership with unclear decision-making processes, informed by a relatively narrow expert perspective, reinforcing the 'group–think' phenomenon. This also tended to result in the overuse of highly technical language with a narrative that focused on describing the problem rather than defining solutions. This was further exacerbated by unclear policies and communications that limited public engagement with public health measures, at times confusing both public servants and the general public.

These responses were further compounded by an overemphasis on prioritising the economy, with fluctuating messages on saving lives and on ensuring that the health sector did not become overwhelmed. This reasoning sometimes resulted in discriminatory decisions that led to many needless deaths amongst the elderly and the disabled. As the pandemic unfolded, this appeared to be a false dichotomy, and those countries that prioritised people's health and lives in their responses were able to contain the spread of the pandemic with minimal damage to their economies and other sectors such as education (Hasell, 2020). In some situations, the overpoliticisation of the COVID-19 response actively led to the bypassing of existing public health and public sector and local government services, in favour of establishing new private sector responses. At times, in some situations, and due to the sense of urgency required, funding decisions and services were commissioned without due transparency.

In many respects, these responses reflect a lack of sufficient appreciation of risk and preparedness systems, which will be discussed further in chapters together with the means to strengthen preventative systems. It is especially notable that countries that were much more prepared and able to swiftly respond and contain the spread of COVID-19 within their populations, were those that had dealt with epidemics such as SARS or MERS in the previous two decades, and from that experience had developed modern and robust public health systems.

In contrast, some countries in recent years had overseen disinvestment in their public health systems, including their health protection and emergency response services and front-line environmental health workforce. In settings where public health systems and leadership had been dismantled and weakened, the senior advisors chosen to inform that government decisions were more likely to be from academic and clinical backgrounds. This tended to exacerbate the reliance on private sector, scientific, research, and treatments in response to the crisis, rather than focusing upon prevention and drawing upon existing health systems and professional leadership for emergencies including the armed forces, and the public and environmental health workforce.

A further dysfunctional response observed in some settings where the situation seemed to be spiralling out of control was an attempt to regain a sense of control by communicating in an authoritarian style and by applying increasingly draconian measures. In extreme scenarios, these patterns of behaviour in response to the crisis resulted in increased political denial, which fed into populist and nationalist narratives, and in turn contributed to social divisions and unrest. At times, this response was further escalated by misinformation, which acted as a driver for the spread of conspiracy theories, including anti-vaccination messages, and wider social discontent. Subsequently, this was seen to lead to further chaos and social distress, undermined democratic processes, and resulted in the fall of some political leaders. Where these scenarios were predominant, the pandemic was able to spread largely uncontained, resulting in significant death tolls which in turn allowed the emergence of new viral variants, and creating further epidemic waves that extended the harm of the pandemic globally.

In many countries, these dysfunctional responses led to a rise in political populism, which also contributed to the justification of 'vaccine nationalism'. This dynamic can be explained through the balance of 'rights' and 'responsibilities' regarding the public health and pandemic responses described in the diagram below. Some countries have a culture that places an extreme emphasis on the right to individual freedoms, even to the extent that responsibilities to others are seen as irrelevant. It has been within these cultural contexts that the rise in political populism occurred as a reaction to the perceived infringements of individual rights as a consequence of public health measures required to control the pandemic. In contrast, countries and cultures that emphasised mutual responsibilities had a cultural understanding that accepted the need for rapid public health interventions which generally resulted in significantly less deaths and disabilities. In reality, viruses do not recognise individual rights and responsibilities, and the dichotomy of these diverging cultural and

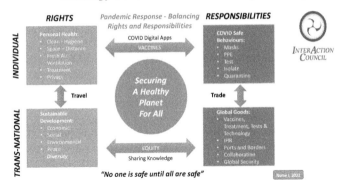

Figure 1.2 Balancing Rights and Responsibilities in Response to the Pandemic

political perspectives is meaningless. However, an appreciation of the alignment of measures according to 'rights' or 'responsibilities' as illustrated in Figure 1.2 can potentially enable leaders to ensure a balance of culturally sensitive interventions that allow diverse communities and nations to work towards common goals (Figure 1.2).

Rather than highlighting failings at individual, national, or global level, this book aims to identify the common patterns that emerged in responding to the pandemic, in order to shape our leadership systems so that we can avert and respond effectively to emergencies of this sort in the future. Devastating as this pandemic was to the global economy, peoples' lives, and global security, the accelerating planetary emergency represents an existential threat to the future of humanity. The leadership lessons from this pandemic are explored in this book to ensure that we do not fail in our collective endeavours to secure the well-being of future generations. The next chapters of this book focus upon understanding why we collectively failed in our response to this pandemic, whilst the latter chapters outline solutions and explore implications for other health threats including the planetary emergency, whilst the final chapters reflect upon how we need to strengthen leadership and global governance mechanisms going forward.

Key Messages

- **The Pandemic – A Failure of Leadership:** collectively, we did not manage to prevent this pandemic, and in many high-income countries there was a slow response by leaders at the outset, which contributed to its escalation at a critical time.
- **Pandemic Imperialism – A Threat to Global Security:** rich countries dominated the pandemic response with vaccine nationalism and a high-risk

approach of allowing COVID-19 to mutate and become endemic, with negative impacts upon low- and middle-income countries, the global economy, and widening inequalities.

- **Expert Led versus Emergency Response:** the health response tended to be driven by academics and clinicians who responded to the pandemic with research and treatments, rather than by emergency planners, public and environmental health professionals who are trained to deal with disease outbreaks and pandemics.
- **An Absence of Architecture for Global Health Security:** although the UN General Assembly and UN Security Council passed supportive resolutions to address the pandemic, aside from the Health Sector response led by the WHO, there was no pre-existing international infrastructure to rapidly coordinate strategic action and galvanise resources at governmental level.
- **The Rise of Nationalism with Rights versus Responsibilities:** across many countries a shift in the political expression towards populism with its emphasis upon nationalism and rights predominated, compared to countries that focused upon responsibilities, negatively affected a multilateral global response to the pandemic.

Bibliography

ABJD Lawyers (2021) 'Complaint before the International Criminal Court' https://mstbrazil.org/sites/default/files/Complaint%20-%20ABJD%20v.%20Jair%20Messias%20Bolsonaro%20-%20ABJD%20ENG.pdf

Ashton J, (2020) *'Blinded by Corona – How the Pandemic Ruined Britain's Health and Wealth and What to Do About It'* Gibson Square Books.

Dyer O, (2021) 'Covid-19: Bolsonaro Should Face Criminal Charges over Brazil's Failed Response, Recommends Inquiry' *BMJ* 375: n2581. doi: 10.1136/bmj.n2581: https://www.bmj.com/content/375/bmj.n2581

Economist (2021) 'What Is the Economic Cost of COVID-19?' https://www.economist.com/finance-and-economics/2021/01/09/what-is-the-economic-cost-of-covid-19

GPMB 2019: Global Preparedness Monitoring Board (2019) 'A World at Risk: Annual Report on Global Preparedness for Health Emergencies' Geneva: World Health Organization.

GPMB 2020 (2020) 'A World in Disorder: Global Preparedness Monitoring Board Annual Report' Geneva: World Health Organization.

GPMB 2021 (2021) 'From Worlds Apart – To a World Prepared: Global Preparedness Monitoring Board Annual Report' Geneva: World Health Organization.

Hasell (2020) 'Which Countries Have Protected Both Health and the Economy in the Pandemic?' Our World in Data: https://ourworldindata.org/covid-health-economy

Horton R, (2020) *'The COVID-19 Catastrophe: What's Gone Wrong and How to Stop it Happening Again'* Polity Books.

InterAction Council (2017) 'Dublin Charter for One Health' https://www.interactioncouncil.org/publications/dublin-charter-one-health

InterAction Council (2020) 'Pandemic Emergency Response to the Coronavirus, COVID-19 Pandemic, Global Responsibilities and an Emergency Framework for Countries and Communities' https://www.interactioncouncil.org/sites/default/files/Global%20Responsibilities%20and%20an%20Emergency%20Framework%20for%20web_0.pdf

InterAction Council (2022) 'Ending the Pandemic: Enhancing Global Security for People and Planet A Framework for the Future' https://www.interactioncouncil.org/sites/default/files/Pandemic%20Exit%20Strategy%20reduced.pdf

InterAction Council Pandemic Recommendations (2021) https://www.interactioncouncil.org/index.php/media-centre/omicron-shows-vaccine-inequality-must-end-says-bertie-ahern-co-chair-interaction

InterAction Council Quotes (2020) 'Council of Former World Leaders Urges Urgent Global Co-operation to Combat Covid-19 and Plan for a Better Future' https://www.interactioncouncil.org/media-centre/council-former-world-leaders-urges-urgent-global-co-operation-combat-covid-19-and-plan

IPPPR (2021) 'COVID-19: Make it the Last Pandemic' Independent Panel for Pandemic Preparedness & Response

Jha P, Brown P E and Ansumana R 'Counting the Global COVID-19 Dead' *The Lancet* 6th May 2022.

NAM (2016) 'The Neglected Dimension of Global Security: A Framework to Counter Infectious Disease Crises' The Commission for a Global Health Risk Framework for the Future; Secretariat-National Academies of Medicine: https://www.who.int/publications/m/item/commission-on-a-global-health-risk-framework-for-the-future

Sachs J D et al, (2022) 'The Lancet Commission on Lessons for the Future from the COVID-19 Pandemic' *The Lancet* 400(10359): P1224–1280.

UK COVID Inquiry - House of Commons Health and Social Care and Science and Technology Committees Coronavirus: Lessons Learned To Date; September 2021.

Wang H, Paulson K R, Pease S A et al, (2022) 'Estimating Excess Mortality Due to the COVID-19 Pandemic: A Systematic Analysis of COVID-19-related Mortality, 2020–21' *Lancet* 399: 1513–1536.

WHO COVID-19 Dashboard: https://covid19.who.int/; https://www.who.int/publications/m/item/weekly-epidemiological-update-on-covid-19---13-july-2022

WHO Timeline of Key Events and Actions in response to COVID accessed 27.01.2021: https://www.who.int/news/item/29-06-2020-covidtimeline

World Bank (2022) Global Economic Prospects: https://www.worldbank.org/en/publication/global-economic-prospects

2 The Pandemic – A Disaster Waiting to Happen?

The history of humanity has been intrinsically shaped by pandemic and plague. Yet in today's world, there is a misguided sense of immunity against pandemics. This view has been especially prevalent within high-income countries, where there is a perception that pandemics mainly affect low- and middle-income countries. Moreover, high-income countries have tended to define the risks of emerging infections and pandemics as coming from low- and middle-income countries. In its turn, this has driven an imperialist approach to Global Health Security, the agenda of which has largely been advanced by high-income countries.

The COVID-19 pandemic, however, turned these assumptions upside down. At its outset, there was a deep sense that this was an infection that had run out of control in China. It was considered that such a thing could not possibly happen in high-income countries with their superior health systems, which significantly affected risk perception and response. Thus, as the pandemic progressed, many of the high-income countries that allowed uncontrolled spread of COVID-19, acted as super-spreaders of new variants around the world. This resulted in tragic consequences with high death tolls in low- and middle-income countries, with an estimate of over 3 million excess deaths in India, mostly related to the Delta variant (Jha et al., 2022). The Delta variant was found to have a mutation similar to that of the earlier Alpha variant (which originated in the UK), which escalated the level of transmissibility of COVID-19 with devastating impacts (Callaway, 2021).

A Pandemic – Not 'If' But 'When'

The false sense of immunity from COVID-19 pandemic felt in many high-income countries, resulted in the ignoring of initial warnings and, significantly, the delaying of responses, which led to the pandemic running out of control within the first few months. The delays in the initial response and subsequent policies allowed a significant spread through the community and can be seen as critical in the lack of effective control of the pandemic. In the longer term, this resulted in a global pathway that destined the virus to become endemic,

DOI: 10.1201/9781003181088-2

with all the risks that entailed, as new variants with unknown impacts continue to emerge. Recent analysis estimates that COVID-19 will potentially take at least five to ten years to reach a more stable endemic state, with new variants causing further pandemic waves (SPI-M-O, 2021). Evolutionary virologists consider that COVID-19 could either become less or more severe. It is not inevitable that the virus will become less harmful over time (Callaway, 2021).

In today's scientific world, how did we fail to predict this pandemic? The reality is that it was considered to be highly likely that a pandemic would occur in the foreseeable future, although, it was difficult to predict exactly when it might occur. In 2017, the World Bank stated that the risk of pandemics had risen over the previous century due to increasing urbanisation, international travel, and demographic growth creating pressures on land use increasing the interaction of zoonotic infections with humans (World Bank, 2018). The United States Intelligence Community, in its annual *Worldwide Threat Assessment* reports of 2017 and 2018, stated that if a related coronavirus were 'to acquire efficient human-to-human transmissibility', it would have 'pandemic potential'.

The 2018 *Worldwide Threat Assessment* also stated that new varieties of microbes that are 'easily transmissible between humans' remained 'a major threat'. In 2019, the first report of the Global Pandemic Monitoring Board, co-chaired by Gro Brundtland, the former Director General of the World Health Organization, that came out just months before the COVID-19 pandemic, highlighted the acute risk of a devastating pandemic (GPMB, 2019). The report described increasing rates of infectious disease outbreaks that had the potential to turn into pandemics, with 1483 epidemic occurrences recorded in 172 countries between 2011 and 2018.

In contrast, the World Economic Forum, which produces an annual Global Risks Report, based upon surveys of business, government, civil society, and leading thinkers, in its response to the Ebola outbreak in 2015 regarded infectious diseases as likely to have a relatively high impact, but with a relatively low likelihood (WEF, 2015). A range of outbreaks of infectious diseases and pandemics including SARS, Swine Flu, MERS, Ebola, and Zika were all relatively well contained, which may well have influenced the lower perception of risk. It was only in the 2021 report, a year into the COVID-19 pandemic that infectious diseases were placed in the upper quadrant of highest risk and impact (WEF, 2021). Many public health experts have highlighted that the occurrence of pandemics is inevitable and should not be seen as mere once-in-a-century or once in a life-time events, which demonstrates how perceptions of risk can be diluted because of the uncertainty of when a pandemic might occur.

How Prepared Were We?

At the World Health Assembly in 2021, the Director General reported that only 70 countries had developed national action plans for health security and that many of these were too underfunded to address critical gaps (WHA, 2021). Many high-income countries thought that they were well prepared, but the rapid escalation of COVID-19 infection made it evident that most countries were insufficiently prepared for a pandemic. Despite the Health Emergencies Program that was established at the World Health Organization (WHO) following the 2014–2016 Ebola crisis in West Africa, the degree of preparedness at global level has also been called into question. Even in 2021, when COVID-19 was well entrenched, only two-thirds of countries reported adequate preparedness scores for the WHO annual review of International Health Regulations (IHR). Moreover, and somewhat shockingly, the Independent Panel for Pandemic Preparedness and Response found no clear association between the Joint External Evaluation (JEE) Scores for pandemic preparedness with national death rates from COVID-19 (IPPPR, 2021).

This reveals fundamental weaknesses in vital preparations. A number of independent reviews on the COVID-19 pandemic revealed that the main focus on pandemic preparedness was for an influenza pandemic. Indeed, the main pandemic framework that the WHO utilised to strengthen national standards was called the 'Pandemic Influenza Preparedness' – PIP – Framework, endorsed by member states in 2011 (WHO, 2011). Even countries that scored highly on pandemic preparedness and considered themselves to be well prepared for pandemics had national plans that assumed that the pandemic would be due to influenza (UK COVID Inquiry, 2021). This gave a false sense of reassurance to countries that thought that they were well prepared. When COVID-19 started to spread, this may have contributed to this false assumption.

Basing preparedness primarily upon the assumption that the anticipated pandemic would be from influenza drove many of the early responses, including the narrative around 'herd immunity' and resulted in the normalisation of policy towards high-risk groups, which were regarded, to a certain degree, as expendable. Thus, policies related to herd immunity as opposed to prevention resulted in many thousands of avoidable deaths especially amongst older people and those with disabilities or chronic health problems. Furthermore, the application of a pandemic plan based upon influenza led to early initiatives that focused upon the development of a vaccine (as vaccine solutions already exist for influenza).

This was a very high-risk strategy that took up considerable resources and effort at the outset of the COVID-19 pandemic when the main emphasis should have been on prevention. For example, in February 2020 the WHO convened a research meeting with 300 experts rather than coordinating global prevention efforts to contain the pandemic. Fortunately, on this occasion, the drive for developing a new vaccine appears to have paid off, but this was not inevitable. There are still no viable vaccines available for many other infectious diseases including HIV and the common cold – both Coronaviruses. Moreover, it could be argued that the amount of time, effort, and resources spent on the vaccine instead of on the basic public health control measures, especially early on, which could have potentially altered the overall course of the pandemic and averted its size and scale.

Chronic Under-Investment in Public Health Systems

A significant contributory factor to the state of poor preparedness for a pandemic in many countries has been chronic under-investment in public health services and systems, including environmental health over recent years. Aside from having a robust plan, robust delivery mechanisms are required to ensure the effectiveness of such preparedness. Such under-investment is likely to have been a significant factor in those countries experiencing proportionally higher rates of COVID-19 deaths. In future, the existence and content of public health operations and services need to be a vital part of the monitoring processes for pandemic preparedness.

For example, a decade ago, the European Regional Office of the WHO undertook an assessment of public health services and capacity across 53 countries and found a lack of a consistent approach to what is meant by public health, including health protection services (WHO Euro, 2012). Further analysis found that the average proportion of the total healthcare budget spent on public health ranged between 3% and 8% with the majority of countries spending between 3% and 5% of their healthcare budgets on prevention (Nurse et al, 2014). More recently, the Director General of the WHO reported that the chronic under-investment in public health contributed to the failings in the COVID-19 pandemic response, with only 3% of Health Budgets spent on promotion and prevention (WHA, 2021). This chronic under-investment has resulted in a range of limitations that were observed across the public health system, ranging from a lack of laboratory capacity for undertaking tests to insufficient capacity at local level to prevent and respond to outbreaks on the ground.

Following SARS many public health services received an increase in funding to ensure populations were protected from pandemic risks. Over the years, however, many public health systems and environmental health services have experienced significant reductions. The Lancet COVID-19 Commission identified strengthening health systems and widening Universal Health Coverage as key recommendations (Sachs et al, 2022). Although public health operations should be considered an intrinsic part of the health system, it is notable that, within the health sector budget, public health services become substantially squeezed and are often seen as a soft target for cuts. Moreover, environmental health and other public health operations sometimes receive funding from other sectors. Protected funding streams must be regarded as a vital element in protecting populations from future pandemics (Figure 2.1).

Importantly, during the pandemic, this chronic under-investment in public health was seen to negatively affect the credibility, quality, and number of

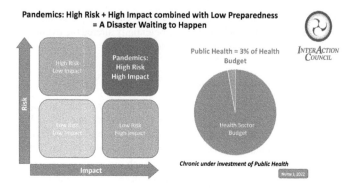

Figure 2.1 Pandemics – A Disaster Waiting to Happen

public health leaders with the capabilities to effectively respond to the emergency. In some scenarios, this resulted in the pandemic response being taken over by clinical leaders, many of whom had little training or experience in dealing with public health emergencies. This tended to produce a focus on treatments and an academic response, rather than on one based on tried and tested measures for prevention that utilised the existing, though depleted, public health and emergency services. In some countries, the predominance of this clinical and academic approach to the pandemic tended to reinforce the weaknesses of existing public health services and capacity. Academics with a clinical background have tended to focus on healthcare and treatment measures as their main response to the pandemic, with their main emphasis on prevention focusing on vaccinations, rather than on utilising established public health control measures. This perspective was further reinforced by the creation of largely academic advisory groups to inform policies relating to the pandemic, to the relative exclusion of those with experience in environmental health and in managing public health emergencies. This further exaggerated a narrow 'group-think' approach to the pandemic response (Ashton, 2020).

Limitations of the International Health Regulations

The IHR consist of a legal framework that requires the 196 member states to monitor and report health threats that are a risk to other countries to the WHO. The regulations mainly focus upon the responsibilities of individual member states rather than international roles and global governance. The IHR has a long history, with an initial International Sanitary Convention established in 1892 to control Cholera outbreaks across Europe. This influenced the development of the International Sanitary Regulations that were adopted by countries at the time of the foundation of the WHO in 1951. Further revisions were made in 1969, to cover five other major diseases – smallpox, plague, relapsing fever, typhus, and yellow fever. Minor revisions were made across the decades, and in 2005 major revisions were developed in response to the 2003 SARS outbreak, which came into force in 2007 (Tonti, 2020).

Over time, the IHR has responded to changes in global health risks and currently has the ability to coordinate public health threats, whilst ensuring human rights and reducing disruption to international trade and travel. Its overall strength is that it provides an existing structure as an international legal framework for countries to protect themselves and each other from health threats. The IHR 2005 currently covers risks from infectious diseases including those from zoonotic origins, and concerns related to food safety, as well as threats from nuclear, chemical, and biological incidents (IHR, 2005). However, such recent outbreaks, including those of Ebola and the COVID-19 pandemic have revealed substantial weaknesses in the IHR, including the reluctance on member states to report an outbreak to the WHO due to concerns about its economic impact upon trade and travel.

For example, the South Africa Government has bitterly criticised foreign governments for their initial imposition of strict travel bans from the region after the official announcements concerning the Omicron variant. A statement by the South African foreign ministry strongly criticised the travel bans. 'Excellent science should be applauded and not punished'. The bans were 'akin to punishing South Africa for its advanced genomic sequencing and the ability to detect new variants quicker'. The statement added that the reaction had been completely different when new variants were discovered elsewhere in the world (BBC, 2021). At the outset of several new outbreaks, the danger of a negative response has led to delays in national reporting. This has occurred at a critical time for controlling an outbreak with the potential to become a pandemic.

Further delays are inherent within the current structure for delivering the IHR, especially at the stage of decision-making regarding whether the health threat is deemed to be a 'Public Health Emergency of International Concern' (PHEIC). The system is that, following the reporting of a threat by a member state, the Director General of the WHO convenes its Emergency Response Framework (ERF) to determine whether the risk constitutes a PHEIC. Amongst the criteria for such a decision are that the outbreak is regarded as a risk to other member states through its spread internationally and that it constitutes an extraordinary event that requires a coordinated international response. An analysis of the process of declaring PHEICs on nine occasions revealed a lack of consistency or transparency, and contradictions about how such decisions were reached (Mullen et al, 2020). On occasions, the process has resulted in delays in taking swift action. Often, the Director General has convened repeated meetings due to unclear conclusions before an independent decision is made as to whether to call a PHEIC. Furthermore, the overly technical language in the communications from these expert meetings has caused confusion and delayed actions amongst policymakers and politicians.

For example, the Director General only declared the COVID-19 PHEIC a pandemic over five weeks after the ERF had been called, due to delays in national and international responses (Chatham House, 2020).

Aside from the delays inherent in the existing mechanisms and the need to develop a swifter response to emerging health threats in order to keep pace with the rapid spread of many public health emergencies, there are a number of other issues that need to be addressed within the current IHR. Calling a PHEIC allows the WHO to coordinate an international response, but its ability to coordinate a meaningful response to the COVID-19 pandemic has been disappointingly absent (Sachs et al, 2022). Although the IHR legal framework requires individual member states to monitor and report annually upon health threats that might affect other countries, compliance for this process has been patchy. Only two-thirds of member countries have reported compliance with core competencies through the WHO's State Parties Self-Assessment Annual Reporting (SPAR) Tool. Moreover, there is no independent quality assurance process, the current system relies on self-reporting. Although around half of the member states have undertaken a voluntary JEE, assessment for the implementation of the IHR, this relies on goodwill and collaboration (IPPPR, 2021). As we have seen, many countries have chronically underfunded their public health services that constitute some of the essential operations required to fulfil their IHR obligations.

Furthermore, many low- and middle-income countries have seen the IHR as an agenda largely driven by high-income countries in order to protect their populations from poverty-related diseases. These have been regarded as neo-colonial demands, with an over-emphasis on compliance to the IHR, at the cost of not providing the basic and essential public health services for the majority of other diseases and threats to health that are not considered a risk to other countries. Designing health systems that incorporate essential public health measures to strengthen cost-effective prevention and protection functions as part of a wider public health service that includes the IHR competencies has the potential to ensure a longer-term, sustainable, and robust response. This will be discussed further in Chapter 6. Current discussions of revisions to the IHR taking place in parallel with the development of a Pandemic Treaty will need to take account of and rectify these existing weaknesses.

Independent Reviews and Recommendations

Prior to the COVID-19 pandemic, there were a number of international and independent reviews which made recommendations for preventing pandemics and health threats, including the InterAction Council Dublin Charter for One Health and the Global Preparedness Monitoring Board (GPMB, 2019), as well as policy think tanks such as Chatham House. These reports highlighted the continued risks from threats to health, the need to enhance governance and financing, and courageous leadership to ensure a multi-sector approach to strengthen health systems. They included environmental and animal health and emphasised the importance of independent monitoring and accountability. A plethora of further independent reviews have emerged since the outset of COVID-19, which have drawn upon and reinforced the recommendations of previous reviews. The diagram below provides a summary of the main messages that have emerged from key reviews, including the Global Pandemic Monitoring Board annual reports of 2019, 2020, and 2021 and the Independent Panel for Pandemic Preparedness and Response of 2021 (Figure 2.2).

The main recommendations can be placed under two headings: governance and public health systems. From an operational perspective, what is needed to strengthen our public health systems is already known. The issue will be further discussed in Chapter 6. For governance, of note is the recommendation to establish a permanent body chaired by Heads of Government or officials of similar standing. This would fill a significant gap on issues of health security within the international community. With the support of the WHO, such a Council could report on risks and coordinate and communicate responses to international health threats. A panel or Council of this sort could also have a role in facilitating independent monitoring and reporting for the IHR and when it is finalised, the Pandemic Treaty. The IPPPR in particular recommends the creation of a 'Global Health Threats Council' to provide an inclusive and authoritative voice to engage political leaders. A Council of this sort could ensure the overall vision of preventing pandemics, through a coordinated response at all levels enabled by financing and accountability mechanisms (IPPPR, 2021).

Unfortunately, progress has been slow thus far in strengthening governance mechanisms, with a series of Pandemic Summits that mostly focused upon the operational issues for addressing the COVID-19 pandemic including financing and vaccination. Over the coming years, the development of the Pandemic Treaty together with further revisions to the IHR will provide a key opportunity to further define the legal framework, roles, and responsibilities

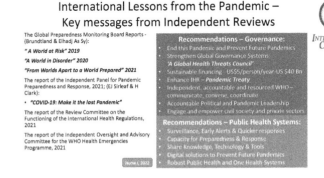

Figure 2.2 Summary of Independent Reviews for the Pandemic

of member states and the WHO. Coordination and accountability mechanisms will be required to strengthen governance for preventing and responding to pandemics. Given the collective failure to deal with the COVID-19 pandemic, mere tweaks to the current system are unlikely to be successful, especially when consideration is taken of the increased risks and threats to health that we face. The next chapter will further explore these critical public health challenges and global health threats in order to inform future discussions on the kind of leadership structures needed to secure our future.

Key Messages

- **A Pandemic of High Impact was Inevitable:** but when it might have occurred was less predictable and affected perceptions of risk.
- **We Were Poorly Prepared for a Pandemic:** with plans that were largely orientated towards influenza with inbuilt assumptions on vaccines becoming available.
- **Chronic Under-investment in Public Health Operations Contributed to the Pandemic:** in 2021, only 3% of Health Budgets were spent on Promotion and Prevention.
- **Legal Frameworks for Pandemics were Inadequate:** the IHR – the legal framework for addressing pandemics has evolved over many years and needs further review and alignment with the proposed Pandemic Treaty to improve future responses.
- **Public and Environmental Health Services need Strengthening:** independent reviews recommend strengthening public health systems for pandemic prevention, preparedness, and response.
- **Global Governance for Health Security requires Enhancing:** independent reviews recommend engaging political leaders to prevent and respond rapidly to future pandemics and health threats.

Bibliography

Ashton J, (2020) '*Blinded by Corona – How the Pandemic Ruined Britain's Health and Wealth and What to Do About It*' Gibson Square Books.

BBC (2021) 'Covid: South Africa 'punished' for detecting new Omicron: BBC News, 28 Nov., 2021' https://www.bbc.co.uk/news/world-59442129

Callaway E, (2021) 'Beyond Omicron: What's Next for COVID's Viral Evolution' Nature: https://www.nature.com/articles/d41586-021-03619-8

Chatham House (2020) 'Coronavirus: Public Health Emergency or Pandemic – Does Timing Matter?' https://www.chathamhouse.org/2020/05/coronavirus-public-health-emergency-or-pandemic-does-timing-matter

GPMB 2019: Global Preparedness Monitoring Board (2019) 'A World at Risk: Annual Report on Global Preparedness for Health Emergencies' Geneva: World Health Organization.

GPMB 2020 (2020) 'A World in Disorder: Global Preparedness Monitoring Board Annual Report' Geneva: World Health Organization.

GPMB 2021 (2021) 'From Worlds Apart – To a World Prepared: Global Preparedness Monitoring Board Annual Report' Geneva: World Health Organization.

IHR (2005) *'International Health Regulations'* Third Edition, World Health Organization.

IHR History: https://harvardilj.org/2020/04/the-international-health-regulations-the-past-and-the-present-but-what-future/

IPPPR (2021) 'COVID-19: Make It the Last Pandemic' Independent Panel for Pandemic Preparedness & Response.

Jha et al, (2022) 'COVID Mortality in India: National Survey Data and Health Facility Deaths' *Science*, Feb 11; 375(6581): 667–671. doi: 10.1126/science.abm5154. Epub 2022 Jan 6. PMID: 34990216.

Editorial Nature (2022) 'Missing Data Means We'll Probably Never Know How Many People Died of COVID' *Nature* 612: 375: https://www.nature.com/articles/d41586-022-04422-9

Mullen L, Potter C, Gostin L O et al, (2020) 'An Analysis of International Health Regulations Emergency Committees and Public Health Emergency of International Concern Designations' *BMJ Global Health* 5: e002502.

Nurse J, Dorey S, Yao S, Sigfid L, Yfantopolous P, McDaid D, Yfantopolous J and Moreno J M, (2014) 'The Case for Investing in Public Health' WHO Europe: www.euro.who.int/publichealth

Oldstone M, (2020) *'Viruses, Plagues and History – Past, Present and Future'* Oxford University Press.

Politico (2020) 'UN Hosts the World's Weirdest Summit on COVID-19 – Lack of Coordination, Urgency and Money Is Crippling the Global COVID-19 Response' https://www.politico.com/news/2020/12/03/united-nations-coronavirus-summit-442599

Sachs J D et al, (2022) 'The Lancet Commission on Lessons for the Future from the COVID-19 Pandemic' *The Lancet* 400(10359): P1224–1280.

Security Council Reports; Health Crisises: https://www.securitycouncilreport.org/health-crises/

SPI-M-O Consensus Statement on COVID-19; UK SAGE, November 2021 https://assets.publishing.service.gov.uk/government/uploads/system/uploads/attachment_data/file/1038072/S1423_SPI-M-O_Consensus_Statement.pdf

Tonti L, (2020) 'The International Health Regulations: The Past and the Present, But What Future?' *Harvard International Law Journal*: https://harvardilj.org/2020/04/the-international-health-regulations-the-past-and-the-present-but-what-future/

UK COVID Inquiry - House of Commons Health and Social Care and Science and Technology Committees Coronavirus: lessons learned to date; September 2021.

WEF (2015) 'The Global Risks Report' World Economic Forum: https://www3.weforum.org/docs/WEF_Global_Risks_2015_Report15.pdf

WEF (2021) 'The Global Risks Report' World Economic Forum: http://www3.weforum.org/docs/WEF_The_Global_Risks_Report_2021.pdf

WHA (2021) 'Director Generals Speech to the World Health Assembly' WHO: https://www.who.int/director-general/speeches/detail/director-general

WHO (2011) *'Pandemic Influenza Preparedness (PIP)Framework'* World Health Organization.

WHO (2021) 'International Health Regulations Core Capacity and Indicators' https://www.who.int/data/gho

WHO's role during emergencies; Center for Health Security, John Hopkins University: https://www.centerforhealthsecurity.org/resources/COVID-19/COVID-19-fact-sheets/200129-WHOsRole-factsheet.pdf

WHO Euro (2012) 'Review of Public Health Capacities and Services in the European Region' by Jo Nurse, Stephen Dorey, Mary O'Brien, Casimiro Dias, Jordan Scheer, Charmian Møller-Olsen, Maria Ruseva, Jose Martin-Moreno, and Hans Kluge: www.euro.who.int/publichealth

World Bank (2018) 'Operational Framework for Strengthening Human, Animal, and Environmental Public Health Systems at their Interface' http://documents1.worldbank.org/curated/en/703711517234402168/pdf/123023-REVISED-PUBLIC-World-Bank-One-Health-Framework-2018.pdf

'Worldwide Threat Assessment of the US Intelligence Community' Senate Select Committee on Intelligence, May 11th, 2017. Worldwide Threat Assessment - dni.gov 2018: https://www.dni.gov/files/documents/Newsroom/Testimonies/SSCI

3 Past Pandemics and Future Threats to Health, Life, and Existence

During the last few centuries, infectious diseases have determined the outcome of colonisation and conflicts and shaped the current political landscape, as well as determining the successes and failures of specific events. For example, a major reason that the Spanish and Portuguese were able to colonise much of Central and South America was due to the introduction of smallpox and measles by immune Europeans into a non-immune population. Between a third and a half of the native population is estimated to have died as a consequence (Oldstone, 2020). Aside from the devastation and death caused by plagues across these communities, the Europeans were placed in a further position of power as they were perceived by the native peoples to have been protected by their Christian religion (Diamond, 2005).

The slave trade was, in part, driven by the deaths from smallpox and measles across the newly colonised lands as there were not enough workers for the new plantations and Africans were already immune to these infections (Oldstone, 2020). Recent estimates suggest that, prior to 1492, the native population across the Americas was approximately 60 million, in comparison to the European population of 70–88 million. With repeated waves of such new infections as influenza, bubonic plague, smallpox, and measles, by 1600 an estimated 56 million people, amounting to around 90% of the indigenous population, had died. This was equivalent to 10% of the global population and it has been referred to as the 'Great Dying'. It caused such a significant reduction upon indigenous American life and farming practices, that due to reforestation, recent studies have linked the global mini-age experienced during the 1600s to the Great Dying (Koch et al., 2019).

Apart from the devastation that these infections caused across these civilisations, they were also responsible for significantly altering the political and geographical landscape of our world today. For example, Alexander the Great most likely died from Malaria or Typhoid Fever at the age of 33, following which his empire was divided up and disintegrated, whilst a smallpox outbreak amongst American troops during the American Revolution, prevented the take-over of Canada from the British, so changing the course of recent history.

DOI: 10.1201/9781003181088-3

A Brief History of Pandemics

Throughout history, human civilisation has been significantly shaped by pandemics and plagues. Historically, infectious diseases have been the main cause of death. During the last century, major improvements to public health such as better housing, nutrition and sanitation, as well as better hygiene and the application of antibiotics and immunisation, led to a decline in the impact of communicable diseases (Donaldson and Donaldson, 2000). In low-income countries, communicable diseases still account for over half of deaths, whilst many high-income countries have levels below 5%. From a global perspective, it was only during the 1990s that a major transition took place with non-communicable diseases overtaking communicable diseases as the main source of disease. The majority of communicable diseases occur in early childhood and many are now preventable by the use of vaccines. In 2019, prior to the COVID-19 pandemic, the leading causes of death from specific infectious diseases included tuberculosis, HIV and AIDs, malaria, and measles, whilst collectively diarrhoeal diseases ranked 8th (WHO, 2019).

Historically, hunter-gatherer communities characteristically experienced the infectious diseases that related to their exposure in their environment, including skin, respiratory and gastric diseases, and malaria. Genetic studies of infections in such communities reveal that they tended to have originated and been transmitted from soil or animals to humans. Historic infections tended to be non-communicable or were poorly transmitted between humans and were chronic in nature, such as leprosy and yaws. In contrast, changes in the way of life in agricultural communities over 10,000 years ago, resulted in more crowded living conditions in one location, often with close association with farm animals (Harari, 2011). In turn, this resulted in an increase and a shift in the types of infectious diseases experienced, including influenza, measles, rubella, mumps, whooping cough, cholera, typhoid, and smallpox. This shift in the nature of infectious diseases during agricultural settlement can be characterised as 'crowd diseases'. Typically, they cause acute illness or death, but, once contracted, they confer lifelong immunity (Diamond, 2013).

Crowd diseases often have their origins in animals. Once they have been transmitted to humans, they continue to spread between humans without the need for an animal reservoir. Although many crowd diseases spread rapidly through dense populations, they require a minimum population to spread – measles needs just a few hundred thousand people as a base and interaction from travel or trade to spread to non-immune populations. The acute and rapid nature of these 'new' infections led to the horrors of mass deaths seen in the roving plagues of the middle ages, as well as the Spanish Flu pandemic that caused an estimated 50 million deaths worldwide at the end of World War I. Furthermore, previously unexposed and therefore non-immune populations (such as indigenous and hunter-gatherer communities) have been especially vulnerable to the severe and acute nature of crowd infections (Diamond, 2005).

Chronic infections such as tuberculosis have existed for millennia. It is more infectious than leprosy, to which it is closely related and thrived in the crowded conditions of the industrial revolution. With the rapid urbanisation in modern times and the consequent crowded conditions in many places, the World Health Organization (WHO) reported 1.5 million deaths globally in 2020 from the disease. These conditions together with the expansion of travel worldwide also favoured continuing widespread infection from small-pox, which killed an estimated 300 million people in the 20th century – more than three times the deaths from World Wars I and II combined (Oldstone, 2020). The continued devastation and fear generated by this disease drove the successful campaign for the first total elimination of an infectious disease in human history, with the WHO declaring the world free of smallpox in 1980. Yet, following this global success, a new infection in humans emerged in the form of HIV and AIDS. Although chronic in nature, it has been described as a pandemic. The WHO estimates that a total of 40 million people have now died from HIV. Fortunately, although no vaccine has been discovered for HIV as yet, the development of medical therapies has transformed the risk of mortality and long-term outcomes for millions of infected people.

Pandemic Risks and Future Trends

The 'Spanish Flu' was first recorded in Kansas in March 1918 and spread rapidly to troops fighting in Europe. The name bestowed on the disease derives from newspapers reporting the King of Spain being an early victim. By July 1918, German Commanders reported that influenza was weakening their troops and interrupting supply chains at a critical time in their campaign – and blamed the disease for halting the German advance. The Germans signed the armistice that ended the war on November 11, 2018. Combined with the surge in numbers of healthy recruits from the United States, influenza may have contributed to securing peace. However, the returning troops who were greeted with mass celebrations contributed to the further spread of the infection, creating a devastating wave of death in the autumn of 1918. Tragically, in total 40–60 million lives were lost from the Spanish Flu, more than twice the estimated 15–22 million deaths that occurred during World War I.

Over the next century, the horrors of this influenza pandemic, which especially affects young adults, have contributed to the orientation of pandemic preparedness. Aside from its acute nature and rapid spread, the virus is able to mutate with significant genetic shifts, thus causing further, although much smaller, epidemics in 1933, 1957, 1968, and 1977. A much more lethal influenza virus emerged from poultry markets in Hong Kong in 1997 in the form of 'bird flu' (classed as H5N1), which had a mortality rate of 60% of all infected humans (compared to 3% with the Spanish 'flu'). Fortunately, the mass slaughter of potentially infected birds that act as a reservoir for influenza viruses averted widespread transmission between humans and the possibility of a devastating pandemic, but the risk of a new influenza pandemic or even a re-emergence of a previous one from an animal reservoir (or generated in a laboratory) is still ever-present (Oldstone, 2020).

Viruses have a variety of origins and aside from the potential harms that they can cause through infectious diseases and pandemics, they may also have assisted in the evolution of life. They are present in all life forms including bacteria, plants, insects, and animals and approximately 8% of our DNA consists of viral relics embedded into our genes, some of which have influenced our evolution in positive ways. For example, ancient viral genes within our cells are responsible for communication between nerve cells and assist in our ability to have long-term memory, whilst other viral genes have reduced the maternal immune response that enhances the function of the placenta (Plackett, 2022). Evidence of the evolutionary origins of viruses helps us appreciate the emergence of new viruses, which is often aided by the transmission of viruses between different species. The World Bank estimates that over 70% of new and emerging infections in humans originate from animals. Increasing travel and urbanisation combined with the enhanced proximity of human populations exploiting new environments that expose them to new infections will increase this trend still further (World Bank, 2017).

Over the last 100 years, this trend has been reflected in the changing nature of the infections that have caused epidemics and have pandemic potential. Aside from the constant risk of further pandemics from influenza, we have seen the emergence of a range of different infections that have caused outbreaks of epidemics and, in some cases, pandemics. The COVID-19 virus that caused the recent pandemic is a form of SARS (Severe Acute Respiratory Syndrome). It was first identified in February 2003 and was successfully contained after killing 774 people. A closely related coronavirus was later identified as the Middle East Respiratory Syndrome (MERS), which spread from camels to humans in 2012 causing over 800 deaths. The increasing interaction between people and animals, combined with urban crowding and travel, is producing the emergence and spread of haemorrhagic viruses such as Ebola, Lassa Fever, and Hantavirus. These are spread by direct contact with bodily fluids, with fevers causing internal bleeding and high mortality rates. Additionally, mosquito-transmitted viruses, such as West Nile Virus and Zika, have spread to new territories in the last decade with the consequent risk of ever-greater outreach (Oldstone, 2020).

The risk of further pandemics is now deemed to be even higher than previously. Chatham House has highlighted the increased risk of pandemic spread from rapid urbanisation, global travel, and the potential of unintentional and intentional laboratory escape. Following the COVID-19 pandemic, the Center for Global Development developed models based upon the patterns of epidemic frequency and geographical distribution, which revealed an increase in both the frequency and severity of infectious diseases transmitted to humans from animals. This modelling predicted that there is a 50% chance of another global pandemic as severe as COVID-19 occurring again within the next 25 years. However, these models do not allow for the intentional or accidental release of a virus of pandemic potential, which could be more dangerous due to genetic modification. In many respects, the COVID-19 pandemic may be seen as a 'practice run' for a future pandemic that could be much more serious. Although COVID-19 is becoming increasingly transmissible, it is not as severe as many other existing infections. The risk is that a pandemic emerges that is both highly transmissible and devastating in its impact regarding death, severe illness, and disability. Unfortunately, this risk is not just from evolutionary mutations but is also being generated intentionally within laboratories (Oldstone, 2020).

Increasing Risks from Genetically Modified Pandemics

We have seen how pandemics have presented a significant threat to the existence of human civilisation. An estimated 30–60% of the European population died, especially in urban areas, from the Black Death (bubonic plague) between 1347 and 1353 with further waves occurring every decade for centuries. Even more devastating was the decimation of indigenous populations across the Americas – largely caused by smallpox, measles, and influenza. Although naturally occurring infections and pandemics are unlikely to cause the complete extinction of humanity, there is a growing risk from engineered pandemics (Oldstone, 2020). 'Gain of Function' research, which involves taking a pathogen and mutating it so that has a new aspect, has created vaccine-resistant smallpox, the reconstruction of the Spanish Flu virus, and combined omicron with a more lethal SARS-CoV2 variant. There is still controversy over the origins of COVID-19 in relation to laboratory experiments conducted in Wuhan. Such risks are increasing with more technologies available and laboratories undertaking Gain of Function research in many countries. With variable regulation and safety standards, this poses future considerable risks from intentional or non-intentional release of highly lethal, genetically enhanced infections into human populations (Kaiser, 2022).

Advances in genetic engineering and Gain of Function research mean that they can now be conducted in laboratories around the world. This increases the risks of developing lethal pathogens with enhanced infectivity and transmission that could leak from a laboratory by accident or be released intentionally for biological warfare. Such risks are leading to greater levels of regulation and surveillance in some countries. However, these standards are not applied everywhere. Some national governments or terrorist organisations may be considering the application of this technology to international warfare (Shinomiya et al, 2022). Once such a lethal pathogen is released it may prove difficult to control. Early detection and public health containment measures will be critical to avert devastating impacts. Unfortunately, the inability to respond swiftly to the COVID-19 pandemic calls into question the adequacy of existing global governance and national and regional public health infrastructure.

Beyond Pandemics – Threats from our Planetary Emergency

Recent evidence is raising serious concerns about the potential escalation of the rate of the destabilisation of the earth and ocean systems that had already begun to occur at an annual average global increase of 1.2°C (Spratt and Dunlop, 2022). That Antarctica, the Arctic, and Greenland are experiencing significant melting of glaciers and ice sheets at a rate much faster than modelling had predicted is of great concern. This is due to the North and South Poles experiencing temperature rises around four times the global average. This is a consequence of warming oceans together with increased heat absorption by dark meltwater in comparison with the cooling effect of white ice and snow that reflects the heat from sunlight. Icebergs require cooler conditions to refreeze, so once the polar ice regions have started to melt at the present extent, unless current trends can be reversed, according to historical records, even at today's temperatures the level of our oceans will rise by 5–9 m.

Further evidence is revealing that other parts of the world are starting to change in ways that could escalate the climate crisis (Kemp et al, 2022). This process is often described as exceeding 'Tipping Points' whereby once a temperature threshold has been reached, it tends to escalate until a new steady state is reached (Spratt and Dunlop, 2022). An example of this is the way that ice in a cup will keep melting until it turns into liquid. This is what is happening on a vast scale across our planetary systems. Moreover, the vast expanses of permafrost in land masses adjacent to the North Pole are also starting to warm and melt. As permafrost melts it releases substantial amounts of methane. There are an estimated 1.5 trillion tonnes of carbon equivalent emissions captured under permafrost regions, which is triple the total of all the global warming gases released since 1850.

Furthermore, carbon sinks, which contribute to the absorption of carbon dioxide emissions, are becoming saturated and starting to release carbon emissions back into the atmosphere. Due to deforestation, drying conditions, and wildfires, the Amazon Rainforest, which has acted as a huge carbon sink, is starting to release more carbon emissions than it absorbs. The oceans so far have absorbed 90% of carbon emissions, but, with warming temperatures, they will start to release them back into the atmosphere which will further escalate the warming of the planet (IUCN, 2016). We stand at a dangerous point at which critical thresholds are being exceeded. If existing trends continue, it could lead to cascading rises in temperatures resulting in an unliveable 'hothouse earth' (Lynas, 2020; McGuire, 2022).

This year-on-year increase in emissions makes our ability to deliver on commitments to keep within safe limits increasingly unlikely. Based upon modelling, the current trajectory places us on a critical pathway that could see a rise in temperatures exceeding 2–3°C by the end of this century (UNEP, 2022). This risks a potential further escalation of temperatures of between 2° and 12°C by 2300 (IPCC, 2018). Evidence from existing observations indicates that safe limits for temperature thresholds are already being exceeded (Kemp et al, 2022). This presents substantial risks from cascading temperatures and climate breakdown and ultimately, unless we intervene, the creation of an unliveable world for human civilisation. The Lancet Climate and Health report outlined multiple health vulnerabilities and impacts for humans in the coming decades, including current and short-term increases in injuries, diseases, and deaths (Romanello et al, 2022). Yet the main risk from climate change is its impact upon the very determinants that are required for life and existence – air, water, food, and a place to live.

The Poly-crisis and Multiple Threats to Life and Human Existence

The immediate threats from nuclear war have overshadowed the longer-term catastrophic risks posed by the climate emergency, although humanity has lived with the threat of nuclear obliteration for several generations. An all-out exchange of 4,000 weapons has the potential to kill billions in its initial impact. Such an event would be followed by the creation of an unliveable world that would be 8°C cooler, in which it would not be possible to grow food for four to five years. Even a small regional nuclear war involving 100 nuclear weapons could result in a nuclear winter that could devastate crops and put billions at risk of starvation (Global Priorities Project, 2017). Despite the progress made by non-nuclear proliferation agreements, the threats posed by the recent conflict in Ukraine have escalated risks and substantially threaten human and global security (Jacobs et al, 2022). Hopefully, we can learn from near misses to ensure that safer designs and decision-making processes and a culture of peace can be created at community level (Bellis et al, 2017) combined with an active emphasis on creating the conditions for peace through trust and diplomacy (Sen, 2011).

Existential threats can be considered as risks that have the potential to eliminate human existence, either in its entirety or to such an extent that human populations and their civilisations are not able to recover for millennia. Such threats could come from natural disasters such as volcanoes, pandemics, or cosmic events such as asteroids colliding with the Earth. However, in today's world, we are exposed to increasing threats from devastation created by humanity itself, including war and the climatic and biological crisis. Furthermore, as technology advances, the risks of either intentionally or unintentionally undermining human civilisation will need to be countered (Rees, 2021). The multiple threats that we face today including pandemics have been described as a 'poly-crisis' of interconnected systems that tend to interact in

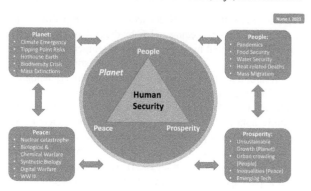

Figure 3.1 The Escalating Nexus of Existential Threats to Humanity

ways that exacerbate these risks (Nurse, 2023). For example, the warming world increases infectious diseases and pandemic risks, whilst droughts drive migration and the potential for conflicts. These multiple links are illustrated in the diagram on 'The Escalating Nexus of Existential Threats to Humanity' (Figure 3.1).

Threats to Life on Earth – Symptoms of a Sick Planet?

In many respects, the threats to human life as well as that of many of our fellow life forms within the context of our biosphere can be seen as symptoms of a sick planet. Given the evolutionary origins of humans from our Earth's ecosystems, analogies can be made between a critically ill person and an urgently sick planet (IAC, 2019). The Earth's rising temperatures can be seen as the development of a fever, which for humans can be lethal even with an increase in global temperatures of 3–4°C. The world's oceans and water systems represent our cardiovascular system, which is becoming increasingly acidic, with the circulatory disruption of our ocean currents. Whilst, the lungs of our Planet are starting to fail as our forests are destroyed, and as we deplete our soils, our skin can be seen to become eroded. Our immune system is reacting to the emergence of increasing pandemics, mass migration, and conflicts. These are symptoms of extreme mental and physical stress, with the beginnings of multi-organ failure and shock. If the Planet were a human being, it would be sent straight to intensive care for emergency treatment. These are illustrated in the diagram below, 'Symptoms of a Sick Planet' (Figure 3.2).

Although an analogy, this comparison can help us reframe the scale and speed of the response required to address the increasing combination of existential threats that humanity faces. The relative lack of acknowledgement or response of these threats within the international community is a matter of great concern. The risks posed by climate 'Tipping Points' are not adequately reflected within current IPCC recommendations (Spratt and Dunlop, 2022).

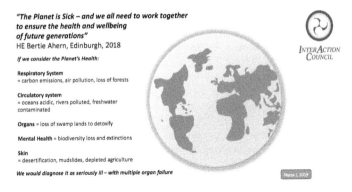

Figure 3.2 Symptoms of a Sick Planet

Having a greater risk analysis, appreciating the interconnections between these threats and taking a coordinated approach globally to prevent, mitigate, and prepare for these risks will be critical for our very survival, as will the application of research and technology to achieve rapid and appropriate solutions (Ord, 2020). We need to apply the lessons learnt from our failings in response to the COVID-19 pandemic, ranging from a lack of risk perception, preparedness, and denial. These are the subject of the next chapter.

Recommendations – Action for One Health

The actions below are recommended by the InterAction Council Dublin Charter for One Health (IAC, 2017), an approach that recognises the interconnectivity between the health of humans, animals, the environment, and the planet.

1 Coordinated local, national, multilateral, and global solutions are required to tackle poverty, global environmental change, peace and justice, access to clean water, and responsible production and consumption.
2 Increased resilience is needed to respond to emerging threats and to tackle the driving forces of environmental change in order to enhance the integrity of the natural systems on which humanity depends.
3 Environmental health should be integrated into health budgeting with a preventive approach. There is an obligation to expand trans-disciplinary research to address gaps in knowledge through defining the links between health and environmental change and to develop potential adaption strategies for populations subject to environmental change.
4 There is an imperative that governance, accountability, monitoring, and independent evaluation be improved and policy, legislative and regulatory changes will be necessary in all sectors related to health – social, economic, and environmental determinants and patterns of international commerce, trade, finance, advertising, culture, and communications.

5   Fearless leadership is needed, as well as whole societal engagement, recognising that governments acting alone will not be able to deliver One Health and will require broader leadership from civil society, the scientific community, academia, local government, and the private sector supported by a global learning network.

6   Establish an independent accountability mechanism to ensure monitoring and review of the aforementioned Actions for One Health.

In addition to these recommendations, further emphasis is required on risk analysis and early intervention, based upon learning from the COVID-19 pandemic and evidence from cascading tipping points. Concerns regarding the exceeding of critical thresholds for safe climate limits and calls to revisit safe thresholds must be addressed. Such a programme will potentially enable the rapid stabilisation of the planetary system to create a healthy world that is compatible with human life and civilisation.

Bibliography

Bellis M A, Hardcastle K, Hughes K, Wood S and Nurse J, (2017) 'Preventing Violence, Promoting Peace: A Policy Toolkit for Preventing Interpersonal, Collective and Extremist Violence' Public Health Wales and the Commonwealth Secretariat: www.thecommonwealth-healthhub.net

Center for Global Development (2021) 'The Next Pandemic Could Come Soon and be Deadlier' https://www.cgdev.org/blog/the-next-pandemic-could-come-soon-and-be-deadlier

Chatham House (2022) 'The Next Pandemic – When Could It Be?' https://www.chathamhouse.org/2022/02/next-pandemic-when-could-it-be

Diamond J, (2005) *'Guns, Germs and Steel – A Short History of Everybody for the Last 13,000 Years'* Vintage.

Diamond J, (2011) *'Collapse – How Societies Choose to Fail or Survive'* Penguin.

Diamond J, (2013) *'The World Until Yesterday'* Penguin.

Donaldson and Donaldson (2000) *'Essential Public Health'* Petroc Press.

Global Priorities Project (2017) 'Existential Risk – Diplomacy and Governance' https://www.fhi.ox.ac.uk/wp-content/uploads/Existential-Risks-2017-01-23.pdf

Harari Y N, (2011) *'Sapiens A Brief History of Humankind'* Penguin.

Hothouse Earth Scenario: http://www.stockholmresilience.org/research/research-news/2018-08-06-planet-at-risk-of-heading-towards-hothouse-earth-state.html

IAC (2017) 'Dublin Charter for One Health' https://www.interactioncouncil.org/publications/dublin-charter-one-health

IAC (2019) 'Manifesto to Secure a Healthy Planet for All – A Call for Emergency Action' The InterAction Council: https://www.interactioncouncil.org/publications/manifesto-secure-healthy-planet-all-call-emergency-action

IPCC (2018) Report on Global Warming of I.5C: https://www.ipcc.ch/site/assets/uploads/sites/2/2018/07/SR15_SPM_High_Res.pdf

IPCC (2022) 'IPCC Sixth Assessment Report' Policy Summary: https://www.ipcc.ch/report/ar6/wg2/

IUCN (2016) 'Explaining Ocean Warming – Causes, Scale, Effects and Consequences' https://portals.iucn.org/library/sites/library/files/ documents/2016-046_0.pdf

Jacobs G (editor) et al, (2022) 'The War in Ukraine – Global Perspectives on Causes and Consequences' Report to the World Academy of Art and Science, CADMUS.

Kaiser J, (2022) 'Making Trouble – US Weighs Crackdown on Experiments that Could Make Viruses More Dangerous' Science: https://www.science.org/content/article/u-s-weighs-crackdown-experiments-could-make-viruses-more-dangerous

Kemp L et al, (2022) 'Climate Endgame: Exploring Catastrophic Climate Change Scenarios' *Proceedings of the National Academy of Sciences/PNAS*, Aug 1; 119: 34.

Koch A et al, (2019) 'Earth System Impacts of the European Arrival and Great Dying in the Americas After 1492' *Quaternary Science Reviews* 207: 13–36.

Lawrence M, Janzwood S and Homer-Dixon T, (2022) 'What Is a Global Polycrisis? And How Is it Different from a Systemic Risk?' Version 2, 2022- 4; Cascade Institute: https://cascadeinstitute.org/technical-paper/what-is-a-global-polycrisis/

Living Planet Report: 2018 Aiming Higher; World Wildlife Fund: https://www.wwf.org.uk/sites/default/files/2018-10/wwfintl_livingplanet_full.pdf

Lynas M, (2020) '*Our Final Warning – Six Degrees of Climate Emergency*' 4th Estate, Harper Collins.

McGuire B, (2022) '*Hothouse Earth – An Inhabitants Guide*' Icon Books.

Nurse J, (2023) '*Human Security and Existential Threats – A Governance Framework for Planet, Peace, People and Prosperity*' Cadmus, World Academy of Art and Science.

Oldstone M, (2020) '*Viruses, Plagues, and History – Past, Present, and Future*' Oxford University Press.

Ord T, (2020) '*The Precipice – Existential Risk and the Future of Humanity*' Bloomsbury Publishing.

Plackett B, (2022) 'Prehistoric Viruses Smuggled Genes into Our DNA' C & EN, Biochemistry: https://cen.acs.org/biological-chemistry/biochemistry/Prehistoric-viruses-smuggled-genes-DNA/100/i15

Rees M, (2021) '*On the Future – Prospects for Humanity*' Princeton.

Romanello M et al, (2022) 'The 2022 Report of the *Lancet* Countdown on health and Climate Change: Health at the Mercy of Fossil Fuels' The Lancet: https://www.thelancet.com/journals/lancet/article/PIIS0140-6736(22)01540-9/fulltext

Sen A ed, (2011) '*Peace and Democratic Society*' The Commonwealth and Open Book Publishers.

Shinomiya N et al, (2022) 'Reconsidering the Need for Gain-of-function Research on Enhanced Potential Pandemic Pathogens in the post-COVID-19 era' *Frontiers in Bioengineering and Biotechnology, Policy and Practice Reviews* 26 August 2022.

Spratt and Dunlop (2022) 'Climate Dominoes – Tipping Point Risks for Critical Climate Systems?' BreakThrough: https://www.breakthroughonline.org.au/climatedominoes

UNDP (2022) 'New Threats to Human Security in the Anthropocene – Demanding Greater Solidarity' https://hdr.undp.org/system/files/documents//srhs2022pdf.pdf

UNEP (2022) 'Emissions Gap Report 2022' https://www.unep.org/resources/emissions-gap-report-2022

WHO (2019) https://www.who.int/news-room/fact-sheets/detail/the-top-10-causes-of-death

World Bank (2017) 'Pandemics: Risks, Impacts and Mitigation' https://pubmed.ncbi.nlm.nih.gov/30212163/

4 Revealing our Hidden Shadows – Emotional Responses to the Pandemic and the Evolution of Leadership

The Pattern of Emotional Responses to the Pandemic

At the outset of the COVID-19 pandemic, a repeated pattern could be seen to be unfolding around the world. Although there were rapid and effective responses in some of the countries that had dealt with SARS across Asia, in the New Year and spring of 2020, many others watched the pandemic expand exponentially in China with minimal response. There appeared to be a general sentiment that the exploding catastrophe would not affect them – and for high-income countries there was the perception that their hospitals were much better than those in China would make the pandemic much more manageable. Furthermore, the global risk perception held a false presumption that led to many national and international organisations to base their pandemic plans upon an influenza outbreak, without fully considering the potential risks from other types of infections.

Many of the evaluations and reports that have emerged since the onset of the pandemic have emphasised the importance of the lost few months of relative inaction at its inception. From a psychological perspective, it seemed that there was a collective denial of the impending disaster. Although some emergency mechanisms were triggered, the sense of urgency was lacking. Instead, Heads of Government went on holiday, and the World Health Organization, rather than going into a full-scale emergency response, convened a large research conference on COVID-19. Many of those who understood the dangers of this public health emergency watched aghast at this relative lack of response. It was only when hospitals became overwhelmed in Italy that many of the neighbouring and high-income countries woke up to the reality of the pandemic, with the growing realisation that this could happen to them next.

In some countries, this led to a rapid shift from sleep-like denial to absolute panic. Having sat watching and doing little for months, within a matter of days politicians went into a full-scale emergency response, but the prevailing panic led to multiple rapid ill-considered decisions, exacerbated by chaotic communications and frequent changes in direction. The panic spread to the general public, many of whom, through a sense of duty – or of fear, responded

DOI: 10.1201/9781003181088-4

to each twist and turn of policy. Others became increasingly sceptical of the chaotic response to the unfolding disaster, which created a lack of confidence and trust in the leadership and an increasing sense of disbelief in information coming from official sources. This, in turn, fed the rise of the conspiracy theories that drove the anti-vaccination movements.

The panic and fear generated by the pandemic created a sense of protectionism, driven by the need to safeguard oneself, the family, and the nation, which further fuelled populist movements and politicians. The increasing populist and nationalist upsurge led to a fragmented global response, which became further exaggerated with the arrival of vaccines and by vaccine nationalism. Although some countries responded in a coordinated and orderly fashion and were able to effectively protect their populations, others went into an overdrive of exaggerated denial of the pandemic and its impacts. Moreover, the response of some political leaders became irrational, ranging from announcements that the pandemic was seen as a sign of weakness, was not that serious, or did not even exist. Unfortunately, these leaders presided over massive excess deaths from COVID-19 across their populations that in turn for many, led to their political downfall.

Although it's a generalisation, these repeated patterns of emotional responses and subsequent behaviour can be understood as part of our human nature and evolution. On a small scale, at community level, many of these behaviours have been protective and given us the evolutionary advantages that will be described in the next sections. This pattern of responses to Threats and Risks, including Denial, Panic, Populism, and Heroism, is captured in this diagram on 'Amplification of Emotional Responses to the Pandemic'.

However, within the context of the globalised world, we can see how many of these responses to the pandemic have become deeply maladaptive, leading to millions of needless deaths as well as economic decline and social disruption. If we are to survive the more significant risks posed by the planetary

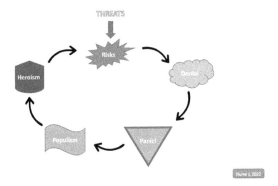

Figure 4.1 Amplification of Emotional Responses to the Pandemic

emergency and related existential threats, we must learn from these failings in order to transform our collective responses to create a safer world. The next sections describe in further detail the origins and significance of these common emotional responses so that we can understand how to transform them for our future survival.

The Survival Cascade and the Response to the Pandemic

The pattern of emotional responses seen across populations and their leaders during the pandemic reflects a common set of behaviours described as the 'Survival Cascade' with the traditional 'Flight or Fight' response to a threat (Mobb et al, 2015). This has its origins within the very foundations of life systems, driven by the evolutionary goal of survival. Observation and research of different species have revealed a common pattern that enables this, consisting of:

- **Fright:** whereby the organism is alerted to a threat. This sometimes creates a startled or hyper-vigilant response, enabling the body to gather sensory details and information to appreciate its nature. It also gives a surge of adrenalin to prepare the body for the following stages if required.
- **Freeze:** movement often attracts a predator and keeping absolutely still helps to reduce attention – camouflage assists further in concealment.
- **Flight:** if keeping still does not work and if feet, wings or a tail are available, then running, flying, or swimming away from the predator as quickly as possible is triggered – some creatures have incorporated a zig-zag response to avoid capture.
- **Fight:** if cornered, trapped, or caught, the creature being attacked often resorts to protective fighting of the predator with the hope of escaping.
- **Fawn:** more recently the 'fawn' response has been described – whereby the creature becomes submissive and makes itself appear cute to appease the predator which may not kill its prey as a consequence.

Fainting sometimes occurs as an overwhelming parasympathetic response that enables a creature to 'play dead' as most predators prefer fresh meat, but sometimes the fear response is so powerful it can actually kill the organism. Although hard-wired into our bodies as automatic responses that bypass conscious thought to enable survival, these patterns vary according to situations. If the predator creeps up on its target without warning, a creature may jump straight to fighting back, whilst a large dominant animal may strike postures to warn a predator against attacking. Not every response is required. If freezing means the predator does not notice it, the animal will move away or resume its activity once it is safe to do so.

Humans also experience this largely automatic response when presented with a threat as animals have evolved with this instinctive survival cascade.

If a person encounters a bear in the woods, the first response is to become aware of and look for the source of danger, whilst keeping absolutely still. If safe to do so, backing away and appearing less threatening is better than running as the bear is likely to give chase. If cornered, posturing aggressively to deter an attack is recommended; and if all else fails, fighting back or playing dead is advised. Although the survival response is largely driven by subconscious physiological reactions, this demonstrates that humans can have some conscious control to avoid danger. For example, we have learnt to jump out of the way of a moving vehicle rather than to freeze like a bunny in the headlights.

Nevertheless, the survival cascade is experienced as an intense emotional response, as the body is flooded by stress hormones such as adrenaline and cortisol, that largely overwhelm our usually slow-thinking processes (Goleman, 1996). Often it is only after the event that the conscious thinking mind starts to interpret and rationalise what has occurred. The survival mechanism has enabled a supremely fast reaction to an immediate threat such as a bear about to attack; however, many of the threats that humans face now are complex and longer-term, and can cause chronic stress and dysfunctional decisions and physical and mental reactions (Harvard, 2020). This interplay of the inherited survival cascade and the generic emotional patterns observed during the pandemic is now described in order to further understand the reactions of individuals, groups, and leaders within a crisis situation.

Risk – FRIGHT: the initial perception of risk in this pandemic can be seen to have been faulty, with a too-narrow framework for risk analysis (only considering pandemics caused by influenza) and a false sense of reassurance regarding the ability to deal with the threat. Yet, once the degree and imminence of the threat was realised, it was possible to observe a fright or startle reaction from some leaders. In contrast, some countries that had experienced more recent outbreaks of disease displayed a more accurate and rapid perception of risk that led to swift actions to control the pandemic within their populations.

Denial – FREEZE: in those countries that were slow to respond to the crisis, there appeared to be a protracted time of denial – either to initially acknowledge the risk or to recognise that the pandemic was affecting their populations. Collectively, nearly two months were lost through the lack of ability to control the pandemic from the outset, as the world appeared frozen in disbelief. The ability of humans to deny impending disaster, tragedy, or death might be seen as a protective psychological mechanism to allow the continuation of day-to-day activities in the hope that the threat is not real, that it will affect others and not them, or that it will simply go away.

Panic – FLIGHT: for some leaders who had initially denied the impact of the pandemic, once the size and scale of the risk were realised, a swift turnaround in perspective occurred. Sometimes, over the course of a weekend or a few days, rapid decisions and plans were put in place, with contradictory messages communicated to the public, that would later be changed, sometimes on that very day. This metaphorical running around like headless chickens, looking for a rapid escape plan, conveyed a real sense of chaos and panic to the wider population.

Populism – FIGHT: furthermore, the rapid and constantly changing decision-making that occurred without any clear rationale led to a sense of fear in the wider population which wanted clear instructions on actions to follow in order to feel safe. The distrust this engendered led to growing conspiracy theory movements with a sense of anger at experts, politicians, and others. With the closure of borders and as vaccines became available, a rapid rush to vaccine nationalism developed, coupled with a rise in populism. Although most people did not resort to violence, considerable anger was demonstrated towards leaders concerning the loss of freedoms, rights, and loved ones. Additionally, people from other groups and countries were increasingly seen as a threat thereby engendering a surge in political populism.

Heroism – FAWN: in response to the crisis, leaders of some countries struck heroic and dominant postures. Such attitudes had their effect in assuring compliance. In most cases, at least initially, people passively obeyed the COVID-19 restrictions that were put in place, despite the impact on their civil liberties. Another manifestation of the appeasement relating to the fawn state could be observed in the significant 'group-think' that occurred across governments and their related institutions. This minimised the expression of differing perspectives that actually could have generated solutions to the crisis.

Unfortunately, although the survival cascade has enabled the survival of animals faced with immediate threats, some of these responses were not helpful in dealing with the pandemic. Such reactions can be seen as a failure to address the more complex and enduring threats that human beings now face. The protracted denial of the level of the threat ensured that valuable time was lost in controlling of the pandemic in its early stages, which could have affected the long-term trajectory and contributed to the millions of deaths. The state of panic observed during the flight stage led to ineffective government policies as well a deep distrust in politicians.

This later negatively influenced compliance with restrictions and vaccine uptake by some sections of the population. The anger expressed during the fight stage was turned against other countries in a growth of nationalist attitudes, at a time when multilateral global efforts were desperately needed. The striking of dominating and heroic attitudes by some senior leaders contributed to the emergence of autocratic and dictatorial political culture. The diagram on 'Emotional Responses to the Pandemic and the Survival Cascade' aligns the patterns of behaviour seen during the pandemic with those that relate to different aspects of the survival cascade.

Understanding the parallels of human behaviour during a crisis with those expressed as a consequence to an existential threat, though not an exact analogy, is helpful in appreciating how responses to further pandemics and threats to human survival may be improved. However, this relationship does not fully

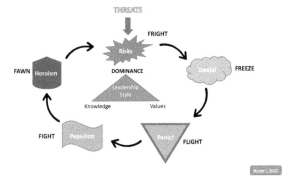

Figure 4.2 Emotional Responses to the Pandemic and the Survival Cascade

explain all the behavioural and emotional patterns that were observed during the COVID-19 pandemic. Although the survival cascade is intrinsically wired into our physiology as animals and as humans, we also have inherited a wide range of other adaptive behaviours. As social animals, it is useful to look at how we coordinate our responses to threats that affect our survival. In order to gain a fuller appreciation of the complex and often subconscious forces that influence our behaviour, the next section will therefore examine the evolution of leadership in our ancestors.

Understanding the Evolutionary Origins of Leadership

Current leadership models tend to draw heavily from a narrow range of human experience, including those from recent history, with a predominance of leadership styles from white, western males, mainly within the context of the private sector. To be able to appreciate the relative failings and successes of leadership during the pandemic, and apply these lessons to the planetary emergency, it is valuable to examine the factors that influence intrinsic leadership qualities. Therefore, this section summarises current understanding of the development of leadership from an evolutionary perspective, drawing upon biological and psychological processes as well as observations from anthropological and non-human behaviour (Garfield et al, 2018).

Approximately 30% of mammals operate within a group, within which the main behavioural purpose of both leaders and followers is the coordination of the activities and social behaviour that provide protection and the solution of problems over competition for resources. Across the animal kingdom, there is a wide range of leadership patterns in order to achieve this purpose. Chickens and cows have a very distinct and linear 'pecking order', whilst the complex and coordinated movements across flocks of birds tend to favour those that are older and more experienced. Wolves operate as a pack, led by an alpha pair, whereby the female leads on the defence and care of the young, whilst the male is responsible for coordinating hunting. In contrast, elephant herds and killer whale pods are led by the older, experienced, and knowledgeable females.

Even across the primate family, which, from an evolutionary perspective, is more closely related to humans, there is considerable diversity in leadership modes. These range from dominant behaviours reinforced by social status to distributed leadership patterns. For example, chimpanzee troops have often been characterised as being led by an alpha male, whilst in reality, social organisation is a dynamic and fluid process. Groups rarely have a long-term leader, and roles vary across male and female chimps according to different functions – such as foraging for food and conflict resolution. Successful chimp leaders exhibit calm and tolerance, are slow to display aggression, and are quick to reconcile after conflicts. Primate leaders develop strong social ties to maintain consensus and harmony, often building upon relationships developed during infancy. Capuchin monkeys display a distributed form of leadership with different members adopting different roles, whilst Bonobo monkeys often have female leaders largely based upon social relationships with minimal aggressive behaviour.

In a similar way, a significant variety of leadership styles has been observed across human history. Small groups of hunter-gatherers tend to have more egalitarian and diffuse leadership patterns, based upon the knowledge and skills that represent cultural values and norms. Leaders within this context are good decision-makers, are relatively extrovert and physically formidable, and serve the collective interest. The larger early agricultural groups that were abundant in resources and were sedentary tended to specialise roles and have ownership of resources, with the creation of elaborate status structures and hierarchies that utilised slaves and widened inequalities.

These non-egalitarian leadership styles were built upon increasing wealth and developing military structures to defend resources. They were reflected by the dominant 'Big Chief' who oversaw an increasingly complex social organisation, which ensured food and protection, and dealt with disputes. In contrast, the more dispersed nomadic pastoralists, largely based upon herding animals and subsistence farming, motivated, and inspired their followers. Their situationally autonomous leadership style was based upon social norms, values, and honour codes. In summary, the main patterns of evolutionary leadership behaviour that have been adopted by humans can be divided into three main areas:

• **Dominance-based Leadership:** based upon wealth, heredity, hierarchy and status, strength, and physical dominance: this style tends to predominate under threats and acts to benefit the defence and protection of the group.

- **Knowledge-based Leadership:** based upon skills and information to coordinate food, shelter, and social organisation, this style tends to emphasise social relationships and consensus-building to deal with conflict – both within the group and by representing the group in external encounters.
- **Values-based Leadership:** underpins decision-making and acts as a force for coherence and motivation for diverse groups of people through the advocacy of principles and values that can be applied flexibly according to the context.

Although these can be seen as distinct leadership patterns, they may have separate evolutionary pathways, and any leader tends to combine a mixture of all these styles. Thus, knowledge- and values-based leaders are generally good decision-makers, with their roles expanding to incorporate the management of rights and the fair distribution of resources, making judgements to punish crime, perform ceremonies, and ensure the care of the sick. Such roles can serve to reinforce their authority. Certain styles can be situational, with dominant leaders tending to emerge when there were increasing threats from which the populace needed protection.

However, as we have seen during the pandemic, dominant leaders can emerge who tend to express counter-productive behaviours such as competition and self-interest. Dominant leaders are also prone to develop the negative qualities that have been described as the 'Dark Leadership Triad' and include manipulative Machiavellian characteristics as well as Narcissism and Psychopathy (Furtner et al, 2017). In contrast, an emphasis on knowledge-based and values-based leadership styles, which tend to serve the interests of the group, was seen as beneficial during the pandemic in controlling COVID-19 as well as minimising wider social and economic harm.

Implications for our Planetary Emergency

The understanding of the evolution of the leadership patterns that have influenced leadership styles is helpful in identifying which behaviour is beneficial for addressing current and future threats and challenges, including the planetary emergency (Figures 4.1, 4.2). Being aware of those innate and subconscious tendencies that reinforce the expression of counter-productive dominance-based leadership styles can assist in building leadership skills that are predominantly based upon a balance of values and knowledge. Appreciating the general expression of the survival cascade and related emotional patterns observed during the pandemic is useful in discerning the hidden and negative influences that drive a population's behaviour, as well as that of its leaders and professionals. Fortunately, a substantial body of work exists that can be applied to controlling emotional cascades and enabling the development of the skills required to reduce the harm caused by counter-productive emotions as well as enhancing the emotional intelligence of leaders (Goleman, 1996, 2003).

It can be argued that relying upon our cumulative inherited leadership behaviour to address the increasingly complex and interactive global challenges is a substantial mismatch of the skills required to tackle such future existential threats as our planetary emergency. Such skills have been developed over millennia in the context of relatively small and coherent groups that protected themselves from external threats, whilst, in today's increasingly globalised world, our very survival will rely upon our ability to act globally, coordinating goods and services and tackling common existential threats together as global citizens. In contrast to the denial observed in response to the climate emergency, a key future skill-set for leaders will be the development of a calm, rational, and scientific response to risk analysis, combined with strong values-based solutions to address the increasingly complex challenges. Human beings are not predestined to be ruled by their emotions. They have the ability to learn, predict risks, plan, and prevent catastrophes. These solutions will be described further in the latter part of this book.

Key Messages

- **Emotional Patterns to the Pandemic:** generic psychological and behavioural responses were observed, including Denial, Panic, Populism, and Heroism.
- **The Survival Cascade and our response to the Pandemic:** parallels with the emotional response to the pandemic can be made with the main stages observed in the Survival Cascade, consisting of: Fright, Freeze, Flight, Fight, and Fawn.
- **Mismatch of the Survival Cascade to Human Threats:** the survival cascade evolved as a consequence of immediate threats to survival, whilst many human threats are longer-term and complex and create a protracted stress response that is not always appropriate to the nature of the threat.
- **The Evolution of Leadership and the Pandemic:** had its origins in the need to coordinate and protect groups and is expressed in three main patterns of leadership styles – dominance-based, knowledge-based and values-based leadership. Countries that successfully controlled the pandemic emphasised knowledge and values over dominance-based styles.
- **Leadership styles Counter-productive to our Complex Challenges:** although dominance-based leadership patterns have been useful for survival when protection is required from a predator or external attack, the emergence of dominance patterns during the pandemic led to increased nationalism which hindered national and global responses.
- **Implications for the Planetary Emergency:** during the pandemic, the intrinsic behavioural patterns expressed by those in leadership positions

were often counter-productive. Having a greater appreciation of our inherited responses can help to create more appropriate leadership skills and systems in the future.

Bibliography

Garfield Z H et al, (2018) 'The Evolutionary Anthropology of Political Leadership' The Leadership Quarterly: https://www.researchgate.net/publication/327825273_ The_evolutionary_anthropology_of_political_leadership

Diamond J, (2014) '*The Third Chimpanzee – on the Evolution and Future of the Human Animal*' Oneworld Publications.

Furtner M et al, (2017) 'Dark Leadership: The Role of Leaders' Dark Triad Personality Traits' Chapter in Clark MG and Gruber CW (Eds) '*Leader Development Deconstructed*' Springer.

Gardner D, (2009) '*Risk – the Science and Politics of Fear*' Virgin Books.

Goleman D, (1996) '*Emotional Intelligence – Why it Can Matter More than IQ*' Bloomsbury.

Goleman D and the Dalai Lama (2003) '*Destructive Emotions and How We Can Overcome Them*' Bloomsbury.

Harari Y N, (2011) '*Sapiens A Brief History of Humankind*' Penguin.

Hardman I, (2022) '*Why We Get the Wrong Politicians*' Atlantic Books.

Harvard Medical School (2020) '*Stress Management- Enhance Your Well-being by Reducing Stress and Building Resilience*' Harvard Health Publishing.

Kahneman D, (2011) '*Thinking Fast and Slow*' Penguin.

Kozlowska K et al, (2015) 'Fear and the Defense Cascade: Clinical Implications and Management' *Harvard Review of Psychiatry*, Jul; 23(4): 263–287.

Marr A, (2012) '*A History of the World*' MacMillan.

Mobbs D et al, (2015) 'The Ecology of Human Fear: Survival Optimization and the Nervous System' *Hypothesis and Theory, Frontiers in Neuroscience*, March 18; 9: 55. Doi: 10.3389/fnins.2015.00055.

Ryder G, (2022) 'The Fawn Response: How Trauma can lead to People Pleasing' Psych Central: https://psychcentral.com/health/fawn-response

Westen D, (2006) '*The Political Brain – the Role of Emotion in Deciding the Fate of the Nation*' Public Affairs.

5 Current Leadership Paradigms – Fit for Purpose?

The Mismatch of Leadership Patterns during the Pandemic

Leadership patterns are inherent to our evolutionary make-up. The main leadership styles recognised today reflect in many respects the intrinsic patterns of dominance, knowledge, and values-based leadership described in the previous chapter. With the advent of the Industrial Revolution and the development of capitalism, a plethora of styles emerged, with a range of theories of what makes a good leader in today's society. The types of leadership styles often included in business administration and leadership training courses are characterised as:

- Autocratic or Coercive Leadership (Dominance based)
- Pacesetting Leadership (Dominance based)
- Authoritative Leadership (Knowledge based)
- Coaching Leadership (Knowledge based)
- Affiliative Leadership (Values based)
- Distributed or Participatory Leadership (Values based)

The focus in the business world is often on enhancing the effective delivery of products or services within a relatively linear field. However, such leadership styles do not reflect what is required to organise or effectively govern multiple services, sectors, systems, communities, or nations. Many such approaches have tended to reinforce power dynamics within dominant leadership styles and focus upon organisational delivery. These were further exaggerated with the emergence of the pandemic, where they tended to result in further distortions of power imbalances, with a greater emphasis on autocratic, authoritative, and pacesetting leadership styles. This in turn was seen to weaken leadership patterns based upon knowledge and values. Aside from having not effectively addressed the pandemic, the mismatch of leadership patterns exhibited during the pandemic contributed to the widening of inequalities and power imbalances.

DOI: 10.1201/9781003181088-5

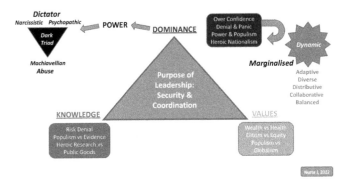

Figure 5.1 Mismatch of Leadership Patterns during the Pandemic

Figure 5.1 highlights the purpose of leadership from an evolutionary perspective as security, protection, and coordination of a group. It describes the counter-productive leadership patterns observed during the pandemic in alignment with the evolutionary patterns of dominance, knowledge, and values outlined in the previous chapter. The rise of these dominant and power-based leadership patterns can be seen to have reinforced the negative attributes of power described as the 'Dark Triad'. In contrast, early successes in some countries in containing the pandemic, often through applying a dynamic form of leadership, were largely marginalised by the increasingly predominant view of the pandemic held by those with disproportionate power on the world stage. The next sections will explore these relationships further to gain understanding on why we largely failed in our response to the pandemic.

Dominant Leadership Styles – A Recipe for Disaster?

Human beings have evolved with a variety of leadership styles inherent in our make-up, consisting of patterns of dominance, knowledge, and values, of which the dominant leadership pattern tends to come to the fore when there are significant threats to security. The emergence of dominant leaders when a group's security is threatened can be seen to have given evolutionary advantage by protecting the survival of the group. During a crisis, the positive attributes of a dominant leader consist of being able to make good decisions quickly and to coordinate rapid action to protect the population. During a war, a competent dominant leader enables the rapid mobilisation of multiple and complex organisations and forces in order to effectively protect the population. This requires a command and control, top-down form of leadership, ideally headed by a calm leader with strategic perspective and sound judgement. During uncertainty or a crisis, many people prefer a dominant leader who is assertive, confident, decisive, and commanding as it provides a greater sense of security and control (Kakkar and Sivanathan, 2017).

Therefore, during the pandemic, it was not surprising to see the emergence of dominant forms of leadership, but such leadership styles take many forms and a dominant style will only be effective if the leader knows what to do in an emergency. Dominating without direction or the right skills and knowledge can result in more catastrophes unfolding, as was observed during the pandemic, allowing its continuing escalation. The expression of dominant leadership styles includes being perceived as confident, assertive, bold, results driven, and commanding, with the ability to make rapid decisions, but dominant leaders can come across as impatient, unemotional, and uncaring. They are often motivated by personal power and can be highly competitive, status orientated, impulsive and intimidating, inflexible, take undue risks, and exhibit poor judgement in decision-making. Additionally, they can be highly authoritative and consider themselves more knowledgeable and superior, taking decisions without consulting others. Dominant leadership styles tend to cultivate a competitive environment that reduces cooperation and collaborative working and can subjugate others to serve their own interests (Kakkar and Sivanathan, 2022).

Although many dominant leaders are perceived as competent, they express attributes that are not always helpful in emergencies, especially when the focus is on protecting the health and well-being of the less fortunate. Although some of the attributes of dominant leadership are helpful for protecting a population from an immediate threat, the range of dominant patterns employed can be counter-productive when dealing with a complex and protracted emergency such as a pandemic. Some of the mismatch of patterns displayed during the pandemic compared to the skills that were required created an unbalanced worldwide hegemony of dominant leadership styles which allowed the further rise of negative traits.

The Relationship of Power, Leadership, and the Dark Triad

A leader is defined by the Cambridge Dictionary as a person in control of a group, country, or situation, whilst leadership is defined as the set of characteristics that make a good leader. The concept of power, which is often seen to be related to leadership, is defined as the ability to command or control people and events. This is further reflected within additional definitions of power that describe influence, control, coercion, potency, strength, energy, and force. However, the word has Latin roots in the noun 'Potentia' that describes having the ability or capacity to do something or get something done, or, of an agency, to be able to modify a situation. The concepts of power and leadership are often intertwined, especially in terms of the dominance styles of leadership. It is useful, however, to separate out these reinforcing concepts. For example, power can be described as a tool, whilst leadership can be seen as a skill-set (Jones and York, 2016). However, the interaction of power with leadership needs to be acknowledged as it can create a reinforcing cycle, whereby its acquisition allows further power to be gained. Research in experimental situations has demonstrated how giving subjects more power lowers their empathy (Bregman, 2020). Unfortunately, as Lord Acton expressed so succinctly: 'Power corrupts; absolute power corrupts absolutely'.

A further distortion of the power seen disproportionately in leaders who are primarily motivated by the acquisition of power is described as the 'Dark Triad'. The characteristics of this terrible threesome are often seen in the career of dictators and warlords like Adolf Hitler. As a crisis allows for the emergence of dominant leaders, the pandemic created an environment that encouraged the expression of Dark Triad characteristics in some leaders. Power drives power, and the pandemic response allowed leaders motivated by power to acquire and express more power. Albeit multi-factorial in its origins, the timing of the conflict generated by Putin's posturing for power within the Ukraine, which occurred two years into the pandemic may be no coincidence. Although consisting of three separate psychological typologies, overlap can occur as a combined triad and act to reinforce the acquisition and maintenance of power. The three aspects of the Dark Triad are characterised as follows (Furtner et al, 2017):

- **Narcissistic Leadership** – consisting of self-centred attention seekers who tend to be arrogant, hierarchical and regard themselves as superior. They are insensitive, lack empathy and come over as grandiose, irrational, inflexible, and amoral; they seek recognition and under stress; and they can become hypersensitive, paranoid, and angry.
- **Machiavellian Leadership** – acquiring power by dishonesty, deceit, and manipulation: abusing their leadership positions for personal gain, perceiving of themselves as superior and others as weak, and utilising rational schemes and tactics to take advantage of and usurp power from others. They are selfish in nature and have poor empathy for others, rarely experience shame and lie to cover another lie.
- **Psychopathic Leadership** – often seen as the most destructive aspect of the triad: driven by power at any cost, they divide and destroy perceived competition and enemies; they score highly on callousness, impulsivity, manipulation, and criminality. Psychopaths seek control and demand conformity and loyalty of followers. They have little empathy and can bully and abuse others.

At the heart of the Dark Triad is a strong motivation to acquire, maintain, and expand personal power. This is often expressed as callousness and frequently related to a lack of empathy for others. All three traits have a disposition towards amoral and antisocial behaviour. Although these characteristics are often expressed in combination, different patterns may be emphasised. Some leaders express their motivation for power through their extrovert personalities, which creates narcissistic tendencies, whilst introverts may primarily acquire their power through Machiavellian tactics. In contrast, the dysfunctional behaviour of the psychopath often has its origins in a childhood that was either abusive or reinforced and rewarded psychopathic tendencies.

The understanding of the emergence and nature of Dark Triad characteristics is important in order that these traits may be identified soon enough to curb, modify, and ideally transform them into a positive expression of power. Many of the characteristics of the Dark Triad have been described as leadership attributes, which illustrates that many of these skills can be re-orientated to mould valuable leaders. For example, some of Gandhi's tactics have been described as Machiavellian, through his use of pragmatic strategies and tactics to gain political support, but these were firmly centred on ethical values rather than on obtaining power for reasons of self-interest. Furthermore, the positive expression of narcissism can include inspiring, charismatic leaders who can positively influence events, build consensus, drive effective performance, create innovation, and potentially shape the future in a positive way (Furtner et al, 2017).

Although only 1% of the population meets the criteria for being psychopathic, an estimated 4% of leaders conform to this definition, with higher rates found in more senior leadership positions, and 12% of CEOs have been found to have psychopathic characteristics (McCullough, 2019). The proportion of inherent psychopathic tendencies is much higher amongst males than females, whether it be related to the achievement of leadership positions or to the number of criminal offences committed, which is likely to be due to a combination of nature, cultural norms, and upbringing. Analyses of childhood factors that predict the risk of psychopathy include selfish behaviour, a lack of empathy, and cruelness to others including animals and are sometimes diagnosed with behavioural disorders in childhood. Such disorders are associated with adverse childhood experiences, such as abuse or neglect, parental conflict, and substance misuse (Bellis et al, 2017). Although these experiences tend to occur more in families experiencing poverty and may help explain why 15% of prisoners are diagnosed as psychopathic. Of course, adverse childhood experiences are also to be found across the wider population.

Leadership positions are disproportionately filled by those from privileged backgrounds, where parenting and schooling may actively encourage competitiveness and status over empathy and values. Interestingly, adult leaders with an antisocial leadership style consisting of narcissism, hyper-competitiveness, and ruthless self-advancement also score highly on fears of compassion, striving to avoid inferiority, fears of being rejected, losing-out or being overlooked, and the avoidance of close relationships (Basran et al, 2019). Although Machiavelli described the manipulative behaviour of politicians as long ago as the 16th century (Machiavelli, 2021), the concept of the

Dark Triad is still a process of being conceptualised, with some authors proposing sadism as a fourth component of an interconnected Dark Tetrad (Bonfa Araujo and Jonason, 2022).

The Marginalisation of Dynamic Leaders

Over-dominant leadership styles have been shown to create a negative culture that reduces collaboration and prevents other forms of leadership from emerging (Kakkar and Sivanathan, 2017). So, although at the outset of the pandemic, a number of countries had leaders that demonstrated a dynamic and effective style of leadership, they tended to be marginalised. Several European and Asian countries, Australia, and New Zealand had leaders (many of whom were women) that reacted quickly to the threat of the pandemic and put in place successful control measures that reduced overall COVID-19 rates, thereby substantially reducing the levels of hospitalisation and overall deaths. They achieved this by having a strong focus on values and placing the protection of people's health as a priority in decision-making. Rather than creating divisions on values driven by either health or wealth, they appreciated the synergies of needing a healthy and secure population to generate wealth. In contrast to countries that focused primarily upon wealth rather than health, the leaders that advanced a dynamic and inclusive perspective that placed people first were shown to have less damage to their economies than those that focused mainly on economic issues (IAC, 2022).

The successful examples of leadership demonstrated at the outset of the pandemic can be described as values based and dynamic in style (Khan, 2021). Aside from a strong focus on people-centred values, they tended to be informed by knowledge, consulting experts, and applying evidence to policy. Their appreciation of the knowledge and skills required meant that many of these countries already had robust plans and services in place having learnt and applied lessons from the earlier SARS pandemic. This led to rapid and coordinated action in response to the pandemic based upon strategic plans and well-prepared public health services. Although some of the attributes of dominant leadership styles were applied to ensure coordinated and fast delivery of protective responses, such styles did not predominate, ensuring a balanced approach across the system. These initially successful approaches can be described as a dynamic form of leadership that is based upon the following characteristics:

- **Adaptive:** decision-making and responses recognising the need to be flexible according to different settings and situations, with the ability to adapt as circumstances change. This is further enabled by having a flexible plan, services, and workforce to adapt to changing requirements.
- **Diverse:** the leadership is diverse and representative. This means that more appropriate decisions tend to be made which take into consideration

the needs of the whole population, including women, younger and older people, and those with disabilities.

- **Distributive:** whereby decisions and power are not held by one person and are disseminated as part of a democratic system that enables active regional and community participation. This style tends to be more consultative and coordinates services and expertise across the system.
- **Collaborative:** a dynamic and balanced style of leadership encourages a culture of collaboration across government, services, and communities, engendering a spirit of all pulling together in a crisis for a common purpose.

Given the early successes of the dynamic and balanced leadership achieved in many countries at the start of the pandemic and, in some, for its entirety, it seems strange that these examples did not cause a wider response. In essence, there were tangible examples of what to do to successfully contain and control the pandemic from the outset. Instead, there was an increasing marginalisation of the successful approaches, which were described as exceptions that were not applicable to what became increasingly the mainstream perspective. Moreover, some successful responses were later blamed and made scapegoats as the cause of the pandemic. Instead, there was the continued reinforcement of the dominant perspective which acted to accumulate personal power (and wealth), for certain leaders, at the cost of pushing other approaches. Apart from denying the opportunity for individual countries to protect their populations, by creating a hegemony of denial, panic, and populism, the predominance of the dominant forms of leadership prevented collaborative efforts to tackle the pandemic globally.

Why Threats Exaggerate Power and Push Away Solutions

So why did certain rich and powerful countries ignore these early successes? And why did dominant leadership paradigms predominate with the consequent responses that allowed millions of people to die needlessly? To gain a fuller appreciation of the dynamics observed during the pandemic and why it led to a failed global response it is helpful to understand some of the intrinsic organisational functions of life systems that create the unwritten rules for how the organisms and organisations of life forms work. This will provide insights into why there is a tightening of control when under stress and why certain groups become marginalised. Human beings are complex animals that have evolved through a multitude of influences over millennia. Thus, it is not surprising that we generally express a mismatch of contradictory and counter-productive responses to challenging situations and do so even more intensely under the pressures of an emergency. Although there is no single expression of leadership, it is helpful to appreciate the hidden influences that drive groups and social organisations, in order to be able to avert disasters and effectively protect populations in future.

Aside from the evolutionary patterns of leadership described earlier, a further perspective to consider is the understanding of the key functions that can be seen as repeating patterns for the organisation of life systems. These reoccurring patterns can be observed across different scales of life systems, ranging from the behaviour of single cells to the evolution of such multi-cellular organisms as plants and animals (Bloom, 2001). These organisational functions have been described as the unwritten rules that influence the operation of such communities of life systems as bees. These patterns are also expressed in how human beings design their communities and operate within them.

The diagram on 'Why Threats Exaggerate Power and Push Away Solutions' Figure 5.2 describes how organisational functions of life systems are recurring operations (adapted from Bloom, 2001), which can be described as:

- **The Centre** – with an inner core of coordinators with a primary role to protect the life system defined by the boundary.
- **Creators and Maintainers** – that provide energy, care, and services to the organism or group.
- **Protectors** – that protect the life system, often with a boundary or wall, a surveillance system, and an 'army' or protective force.
- **Explorers** – that identify sources of food, resources, or energy as well as act as an extended surveillance system identifying distant dangers.
- **Communicators** – enable messages to be transferred between the centre and the exterior of the life system.
- **Healers** – identify, repair, or transform any damage or injury within the life system: includes distant healers that communicate information back to the centre to allow coordinated responses, as seen in immune systems.

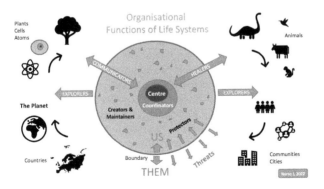

Figure 5.2 Why Threats Exaggerate Power and Push Away Solutions

During the pandemic, the operational functions of life systems can be seen to have been under stress that acted to exaggerate the impact of these operations. Across populations, the pandemic activated a series of psychological mechanisms which are described as the Behaviour Immune System (Bacon and Corr, 2020). This tends to be triggered when there is the threat of a disease and it results in changes to a population's behaviour, including greater conformity to social norms, and a greater aversion to and suspicion of the unfamiliar and outsiders. In essence, it reinforces the sense of 'us versus them' with those inside of the boundary being perceived as insiders, and those on the outside as 'others' and not be trusted. Those on the outside can be treated with suspicion and even be blamed for the threat and become scapegoats.

Although the Behaviour Immune System clearly has advantages in the survival of animal populations – by avoiding other creatures that may be a source of infection and is a mechanism that may have helped protect vulnerable people during the pandemic, some of these behavioural patterns can be seen as counter-productive. In part, it explains the emergence of populism and nationalist responses to protect the group and, in so doing, tends to reinforce the rise of a dominant centre or leader. This process creates a tighter and more cohesive population reinforced by strong central leadership, coordination, and group-think, which actively excludes others with alternative narratives and solutions.

Power, Equity, and Leadership – Everyone's Health Matters

The predominant response of leadership during the pandemic entailed a dominance-based style, which although providing a greater initial sense of protection for the group, generated substantial mismatches of leadership patterns in relation to the skills required to successfully prevent the spread of the pandemic. Dynamic leaders that applied the values and knowledge-based leadership that resulted in swift action and initial successes in preventing the spread of the pandemic became increasingly marginalised and may have been obliged to adopt a response driven by the dominance style leaders, with a subsequent rise in deaths. Many, though not all, leaders who expressed a dynamic style that balanced values with knowledge to inform their decisions were females who became increasingly marginalised by the most dominant male leaders. This illustrates the exaggerated power dynamics that can rise to the fore during an emergency, sometimes framed as the expression of hyper-masculinity. Although it is useful for a group to feel protected and that the leader is in charge during an emergency, this style is only effective if balanced by strong values and informed by knowledge and skills.

The rise of the dominance-based leadership style that became exaggerated during the pandemic can be seen to be a substantial mismatch of evolved leadership patterns to address the increasingly complex and protracted emergencies in the modern world. It is useful for a group to hide behind the biggest and bravest leader when a lion is attacking it, but a pandemic is a very different beast and requires a very different set of skills. The rise of dominant styles of leadership was associated with high rates of death and disability from COVID-19 and can be seen to have been highly counter-productive to the creation of an effective global response. The surge in power, populism, and vaccine nationalism has marginalised small and low- and middle-income countries and widened worldwide inequalities. Aside from the negative impacts this has had on the ability to advance the Sustainable Development Goals, even high-income countries have seen a drop in life expectancy.

The most significant contradiction during the pandemic was the actions of powerful leaders to protect defined populations and nations, in order to maintain privilege, whereas in reality viruses do not respect artificially created borders. Understanding the hidden drivers for human behaviour during a pandemic, as expressed by the Behaviour Immune System within the context of organising principles for groups and life systems is helpful to appreciate how to anticipate and address counter-productive behaviour. During a pandemic, everybody's health matters, and everyone needs to be protected if the pandemic is to be prevented from spreading. Prioritising the vaccination of rich countries creates an illusion of safety, as the more a virus is allowed to spread and evolve, the more opportunities it has to create a mutation that is more dangerous to humans. A full appreciation of the nature of health as a global good means that the boundary for the group or life system needs to be drawn worldwide and not just around certain privileged populations or individual nations.

Key Messages

- **Mismatch of Leadership Patterns:** during the pandemic, dominance-based leadership styles rose in many countries and contributed to the rise of nationalist responses, so reducing the ability to create an effective global response.
- **Dominant Leadership Styles:** evolved to protect groups from attacks and wars and to make people feel safe; however, dominant leaders are mostly driven by power which can lead to counter-productive traits, inequalities, and power imbalances.
- **Power and the Dark Triad:** the rise of dominance-based leadership styles reinforced the authority of authoritarian leaders and dictators with the Dark Triad traits of Narcissism, Machiavellianism, and Psychopathy that are largely driven by power.
- **The Marginalisation of Dynamic Leaders:** the rise of dominance-based leadership styles marginalised dynamic leaders who applied knowledge and values-based leadership to prevent the pandemic and protect their populations.

- **Why Threats Exaggerate Power and Push Away Solutions:** creatures, communities, or countries follow similar patterns with a coordinating centre and a protective boundary: during a threatening situation, the centre is protected with an enhancement of detection of threats from outsiders; this includes rejecting possible solutions and can reinforce insular and populist responses.
- **Everyone's Health Matters:** a pandemic affects everyone and viruses do not respect artificial boundaries, therefore a global response is required and health needs to be seen as a global good whereby everybody's health is protected and valued.

Ultimately, we are not predestined by our biology or our evolutionary drivers. Becoming aware of our hidden motivations will enable us to develop the skills and leadership qualities needed to address future pandemics. For example, the negative association of the term *Fuhrer*, which means 'Leader' in German, has resulted in substantial changes in the concepts and expression of leadership within German culture and illustrates the possibilities of transforming the culture and characteristics of leadership. Ultimately, it is helpful to understand leadership styles and drivers from an evolutionary perspective so that we can respond with a more suitable set of skills for future pandemics and threats to health and life. This understanding needs to be within the context of how groups and life systems organise themselves as part of a complex adaptive system.

Appreciating the mismatch and counter-productive nature of leadership styles in addressing increasingly complex emergencies, including the planetary emergency will be key to our survival as a human species. A greater awareness of which leadership styles fail and succeed in response to our polycrisis and emergency situations will provide the skills and tools required to secure the well-being of future generations. Whilst the first half of this book has examined why we collectively failed in our response to the pandemic, the second half draws upon these lessons in order to identify solutions for improving leaders and leadership mechanisms to prevent future pandemics and reduce the multiple threats to human security, including those from our planetary emergency.

Bibliography

Bacon A M and Corr P J, (2020) 'Behavioural Immune System Responses to Coronavirus: A Reinforcement Sensitivity Theory Explanation of Conformity, Warmth Toward Others and Attitudes Toward Lockdown' *Frontiers in Psychology* 11: 566237. https://doi.org/10.3389/fpsyg.2020.566237.

Basran J et al, (2019) 'Styles of Leadership, Fears of Compassion, and Competing to Avoid Inferiority' *Frontiers in Psychology*, 22 January 2019; https://doi.org/10.3389/fpsyg.2018.02460

Bellis M A, Hardcastle K, Hughes K, Wood S and Nurse J, (2017) 'Preventing Violence, Promoting Peace: A Policy Toolkit for Preventing Interpersonal, Collective and Extremist Violence' Public Health Wales and the Commonwealth Secretariat.

Bloom H, (2001) *'Global Brain – The Evolution of Mass Mind from the Big Bang to the 21st Century'* Wiley.

Bonfa-Araujo B and Jonason P K, (2022) 'Considering Sadism in the Shadow of the Dark Triad Traits: A Meta-Analytic Review of the Dark Tetrad' *Science Direct*, Oct. 197: 111767.

Bregman R, (2020) *'Humankind - A Hopeful History'* Bloomsbury.

Furtner M et al, (2017) 'Dark Leadership: The Role of Leaders' Dark Triad Personality Traits' Chapter in Clark MG and Gruber CW (Eds) *'Leader Development Deconstructed'* Springer.

IAC (2022) 'Ending the Pandemic - Enhancing Global Security for Planet and People, A Framework for the Future' The InterAction Council: https://www.interactioncouncil.org/sites/default/files/Pandemic%20Exit%20Strategy%20reduced.pdf

Jones A M and York S L, (2016) 'The Fragile Balance of Power and Leadership' *The Journal of Values-Based Leadership* 9(2): Article 11: https://scholar.valpo.edu/jvbl/vol9/iss2/11/

Kakkar H and Sivanathan N, (2017) 'Why We Prefer Dominant Leaders in Uncertain Times' Harvard Business Review: https://hbr.org/2017/08/why-we-prefer-dominant-leaders-in-uncertain-times

Kakkar H and Sivanathan N, (2022) 'How Dominant Leaders Go Wrong' Scientific American: https://www.scientificamerican.com/article/how-dominant-leaders-go-wrong/

Khan Z, (2021) *'Dynamic Leadership – A Visionary Leader that Changes the World'* AuthorHouse, UK.

Machiavelli N, (2021) *'Machiavelli: On Politics and Power'* Restless Classics.

McCullough J, (2019) 'The Psychopathic CEO' Forbes: https://www.forbes.com/sites/jackmccullough/2019/12/09/the-psychopathic-ceo/

6 How to Prevent a Pandemic – Prevention and Public Health

Was the COVID-19 Pandemic Preventable?

The first half of this book describes our collective failure in preventing the pandemic, and the reasons why it failed, as well as the risks from future pandemics and global threats to life and health. The points below summarise how we failed to prevent the pandemic:

- **Ignored Risks:** we knew that pandemics were high-risk and high-impact events.
- **Underinvested in Prevention:** we underinvested in public health systems nationally, regionally, and globally, neglecting our insurance system for preventing pandemics.
- **Prepared for the Wrong Thing:** we had a narrow risk perspective and prepared for a different pandemic.
- **Failed to act at a Critical Stage:** many political leaders ignored and denied early alerts and warning signs, which lost valuable time.
- **Reaction versus Prevention:** many countries focused upon suppression and mitigation rather than prevention and elimination which resulted in a poorly contained spread for most countries.
- **Fragmented Responses:** global efforts mostly focused upon raising funds, research, and the creation of vaccines, which widened global inequalities with vaccine nationalism.
- **Lack of Political Leadership:** we lacked substantial political commitment for an international strategic and coordinated response to contain and end the pandemic.
- **National versus Global Responses:** the rise of the populism encouraged by some politicians acted to widen inequalities and made it increasingly difficult to mount a global response.
- **Became Overwhelmed:** allowing the continued spread of COVID-19 created opportunities for the virus to mutate, and resulted in a default policy of 'learning to live with it'.

DOI: 10.1201/9781003181088-6

It is evident that, for the foreseeable future, we will be subject to continued viral mutations and pandemic waves, with the resultant needless deaths and disabilities. Due to faulty policy decisions made by a small number of countries, we are now in a situation where we have no choice but to learn to live with COVID. The reproduction rate at the onset of the pandemic was 2–3. In early 2023, it was 16 as it started to spread rapidly across China with the lifting of their COVID zero policy. The International Monetary Fund estimates that the global costs of the pandemic will be $12.5 trillion by 2024. Aside from the untold personal tragedies that unfolded in many families and communities, long COVID is leaving a trail of disability and economic destruction. We are witnessing the negative play-out of the rise of populism and widening inequalities, with political destabilisations, emerging conflicts, and wars.

Ultimately, the key question is whether the COVID-19 pandemic was preventable, despite all the obstacles and challenges encountered. In essence, if we could go back in history, could we have done things differently in ways that would have prevented the pandemic from occurring, or was it inevitable? Certainly, our leaders want us to believe that it was so and that they did their very best in difficult circumstances. However, this book is not about judging individuals or individual situations, it is about understanding human nature and human systems in order to learn from and adjust our processes to create a safer world.

The Independent Panel for Pandemic Preparedness and Response certainly considers that the COVID-19 pandemic was preventable. In its report 'COVID-19: Make it the Last Pandemic' (IPPPR, 2021), it concluded that the pandemic could indeed have been prevented. However, the multiple gaps, delays, weaknesses, and failures that characterised the whole process meant that prevention did not occur. Fundamentally, it acknowledged that we knew how to stop this pandemic and did not apply existing knowledge at the international or national level. Chronic underinvestment in the WHO and public health systems led to most countries being unprepared and led to variable responses. February 2020 was a critical month with delayed reactions at the outset that could have prevented the pandemic. The report states that global political leadership was absent, and the response resulted in widening inequalities. In retrospect, there were multiple opportunities where the pandemic could have been prevented from either occurring at all or been contained and brought to an end. Key areas are described below.

Key Areas that Could Have Prevented the COVID-19 Pandemic

- **Preparedness:** we could have had a more robust and flexible plan that applied learning from the Sendai Framework with an all-hazards multi-sector approach to addressing pandemics. This could have included a strong emphasis on resilience, surveillance, detection, early warning systems, and early responses with a drive for containment, elimination, and minimisation of harm.

- **Communication of Risks and Alerts:** valuable time was lost at the beginning of the pandemic. Rapid international alerts with objective decision-making processes are required, combined with clear communications in non-technical language aimed at politicians and policymakers.
- **Global Strategic Ambition:** a handful of national and international leaders and organisations could have changed the default of 'learning to live with it' by advocating and investing in a global elimination or exit strategy for the pandemic – this would have been especially effective earlier on in the pandemic.
- **Global Coordination:** the UN system and the WHO could potentially have mobilised political commitment and health sector activities with a focus on eliminating the pandemic and creating an effective exit strategy.
- **Creation of Global Goods:** vaccine research, production, and roll-out could have been achieved equitably, efficiently, and effectively if they had been created and delivered as 'global goods' whose benefits affect all the world's peoples. This could also have encompassed tests, protective equipment, and medical treatments.
- **Robust Public Health Systems:** if adequate services and capacity had been invested into international, national, and community public health systems, the pandemic could have been averted. This could potentially have been achieved by a shift from an average of 3–5% invested into public health services and capacity as part of the health sector budget.

Additionally, there are more upstream areas that could have prevented the pandemic, including greater governance for animal health including that for wild animals and wet markets. After a few years, disinvestment occurred on research into SARS. In future, research on those infections with pandemic potential needs to be prioritised. Critically, pandemics require a swift and coordinated global response. Current international processes, including the International Health Regulations (IHRs), tend to reinforce national responses (Wenham et al, 2022). As it stands, the proposed Pandemic Treaty is unlikely to create a sufficiently robust system to prevent future pandemics.

The next sections describe the importance of prevention and outline how this can be achieved through robust public health operations as a core component of the health system. Global coordination and governance mechanisms are discussed later in the book.

Prevention – A Critical Concept

The COVID-19 pandemic could have been prevented. Independent reviews have concluded that it could have been stopped at various stages in the response. Since its outset, several outbreaks of epidemics that had pandemic potential have been prevented. All were prevented early, due to rapid, coordinated responses combined with community engagement. We know that prevention works, and we know the methods to make it work.

The concept of prevention when practically applied to pandemics can make a critical difference to the outcome. Ideally, they are prevented in the early stages to ensure that they never actually become a pandemic. This clearly is the approach that results in the least harm to health, society, and the economy. Preventing a pandemic from occurring in the first place requires the identification of risks, surveillance of these risks, with early alert systems and rapid containment measures. Early prevention can involve the modification of risk factors, by promoting healthy animal welfare and protecting environments and habitats to reduce the risk of spill-over of infections from animals to humans. For many, the term prevention provides a reassuring message with popular appeal. However, its meaning is used differently in a variety of contexts and professional backgrounds. From a public health perspective, the term is described below in relation to the prevention of pandemics:

Primary Prevention – whereby the onset of a pandemic is prevented from occurring in the first place:

- **Reduce Animal Spill-Over:** including the protection of high-risk environments, healthy animal husbandry, governance of animal and wet markets, and the sale of wild meat.
- **International Governance and Controls for Synthetic Pandemics:** of knowledge and materials for the development of genetically engineered infections.
- **Identification of High-Risk Situations:** to build resilient and healthy populations, environments, and systems; monitor regularly for early signs of risk of infection.
- **Identify and Intervene Early:** enhance surveillance, early detection, and alerts to intervene at the outset.

Secondary Prevention – early detection with early intervention applied to halt and reverse progression of a potential pandemic:

- **Reduce Spread between Countries and Communities:** containment, quarantine, and limit travel
- **Reduce Community Spread:** implement public health measures, such as social distancing, ventilation, hygiene, face coverings, and community lockdowns
- **Protect High-Risk Populations:** through enhanced public health measures such as Personal Protective Equipment, with social and economic support

Tertiary Prevention – to make an established problem less severe in order to improve outcomes; this includes treatment to mitigate impacts:

- **Vaccination: If Possible and Available:** develop and deliver at scale, vaccinations to protect populations – the process needs to be managed as a common good to ensure vaccine equity in order to reduce global spread with mutations and prevent repeat pandemics from occurring.
- **Medical Management and Clinical Treatments:** for infected and unwell people, including oxygen, medications, and healthcare treatment including intensive care units, that reduce the severity of the disease, disability, and deaths.

Quaternary Prevention: rehabilitation and recovery of individuals, communities, and countries following a pandemic. Research and evaluation on the pandemic and the response in order to improve future capacity, services, processes, and interventions. Enhance resilience to improve the population's health and the responses for future pandemics.

Learn from Success to Prevent Future Pandemics

Even when the pandemic had taken hold, we had the opportunity to bring it to an end. Early on there were a number of countries that successfully controlled the pandemic within their own communities, resulting in minimal deaths. During the first year, public health professionals called for an elimination strategy, which is generally seen as the desirable response to the emergence of a new infection (Baker et al, 2020). A review of over 100 articles on exit strategies found similarities in effective approaches. These consisted of implementing the strategy during the post-peak period with a controlled and step-by-step flexible plan, informed by surveillance. Effective exit strategies maintained a continuation of public health measures, including social distancing, face masks, and hygiene measures in combination with vaccination. In contrast, repeated lockdowns or hard exits had limited effectiveness (Misra et al, 2022). Better outcomes for health, the economy, and civil liberties were found with elimination strategies compared to mitigation measures in the first year of the pandemic. During the second year, an elimination strategy was still potentially possible with the emergence of vaccines; to achieve this would have required global coordination and equitable dissemination (Oliu-Barton et al, 2022).

Approximately half the nations of the world created a COVID-19 App to enable contact tracing, provide alerts, and convey public health messages. In the future, there will be opportunities to create a global ready-made flexible app that could be adapted to each country's requirements (P4PPP, 2022). This would allow a rapid and coordinated global response, especially if anonymous data were shared on a digital platform to facilitate strategic and targeted action. It would also provide consistent and responsive approaches that enabled trade and travel during a future pandemic. The pandemic saw a major shift to the adoption of online working which created efficiencies and continues

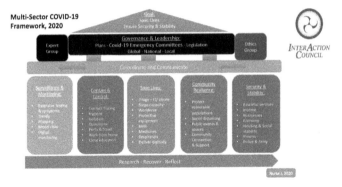

Figure 6.1 The Emergency Framework for Countries and Communities for COVID-19

to transform how many services, including health, are now delivered. In the future, with the emergence of quantum computing and artificial intelligence, there will be considerable opportunities to expand the role of digital solutions for pandemics. Existing digital solutions that could be scaled up to prevent future pandemics include surveillance, mapping of risks and geographical spread, alert systems, communications, coordination, testing, contact tracing, travel and quarantine, and clinical management tools (P4PPP, 2022).

There have been many countries that have managed to control the spread of COVID-19 within their populations, and in some cases, they avoided extensive lockdowns and allowed the continuation of economic and social activities. Drawing upon successful responses to the COVID-19 pandemic from around the world, an overarching Emergency Framework was created to enable a flexible and tailored response within different community or national settings. Figure 6.1 was produced by the InterAction Council in consultation with international Public Health and professional organisations and endorsed by a range of leadership and advocacy bodies (IAC, 2020).

This multi-sector framework is built upon core public health operations and early examples of good practice from a range of settings. The framework provides a visual summary that captures key aspects of successful responses that contained the spread of COVID-19, as outlined in the InterAction Council report of 2020 and summarised below:

Summary of Good Practice during the Pandemic (IAC, 2020):

Act Swiftly: convene emergency committees to oversee strategic plans and exit strategies.

Communicate and Coordinate: ensure clear lines of co-ordination between sectors and geographical levels, and establish daily communications supported by social media.

Stop the Spread: prevent transmission with **enhanced testing and isolation of infected cases and their contacts**, and public health measures.

- **Social Distancing** – of two metres plus.
- **Constant Cleaning** – hands and touch surfaces.
- **Maintain Masks** – indoors and for crowded spaces.
- **Reduce Social Mixing** – between households and communities.
- **Restrict Travel** – plus test and quarantine at borders.
- **Interact Outdoors or Online** – for work and education.
- **Stay at Home** – and shield vulnerable groups.

Vaccinate at Speed and Scale: especially targeting high-risk populations, sharing and expanding supplies, and organising vaccination campaigns through existing mechanisms including Community Health Services, Local Government, Volunteer networks, and the Military.

Enable Health Services to Save Lives: with a surge in the capacity of the health sector and triage systems, redeployment of staff: buildings to be supplied with protective equipment, beds, and respirators; regularly test and vaccinate frontline workers to ensure their safety and to maintain a sufficient workforce.

Enhance Community Resilience, Security, and Stability: target and protect vulnerable populations; stabilise economic impacts; and ensure essential services and wider security.

Research, Recover and Reflect: fast track research, establish Recovery Committees for long-term planning; evaluate and reflect to improve emergency responses in the future.

Prevention and Protection – Core Components of the Health System

Effective responses to the pandemic were rapidly established in countries that had recently modernised their public health functions, services, and workforce, often in response to controlling SARS, Ebola, or Polio. Robust services and a well-trained workforce as part of a public health system are needed to prevent pandemics. Community frontline specialists are critical in the fields of Environmental and Public Health for early prevention measures to be effective. To raise expertise in a workforce, public health operations are best embedded within health systems as well as emergency response processes. National and international strategic public health leaders familiar with dealing with population-wide emergencies are required to ensure robust preparedness plans and response systems are in place and incorporated into mainstream emergency operations to enable responses to emergencies at short notice.

Unfortunately, even after 70 years, the World Health Organization still has no clear concept of what essential public health functions are (WHO, 2018). Although most of its regions have created their own sets of essential public health functions and operations, there is no established central consensus. The WHO Health Systems Framework and Programme has mainly focused on Universal Health Coverage for hospitals and medical treatments, with public health services and capacity largely absent from its resources, publications, and indicators. Somewhat belatedly, during the pandemic, the WHO released a position paper on 'Building Health Systems resilience for Universal Health Coverage and Health Security during the COVID-19 Pandemic and Beyond' which included a recommendation to invest in essential public health functions, including those needed for all-hazards emergency risk management (WHO, 2021).

In the absence of the WHO leading on strengthening essential public health operations, including how these can be delivered within services as part of the wider health and security systems, the World Federation of Public Health Associations (WFPHA) has published a framework. This came about from a WFPHA working group and built upon a review of regional Essential Public Health Operations and Functions, and consultations with key public health bodies including the WHO, to establish a 'Global Charter for the Public's Health' (WFPHA, 2016). As a key architect of this framework, the author, as Head of Health for the Commonwealth, and in partnership with the WFPHA, incorporated the Charter across the 'Systems Framework for Healthy Policy, an implementation tool of the Charter for the Public's Health' (Commonwealth, 2016). This aimed to embed public health operations throughout the health system, and in so doing, create an effective, efficient, and sustainable system as part of Universal Health Coverage. Figure 6.2 describes the main components, of which protection can be seen as an essential public health operation.

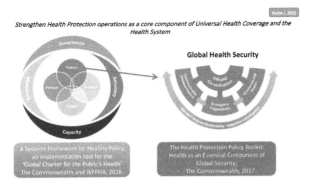

Figure 6.2 Mainstream Essential Public Health Operations, including Health Protection within the Health System

Components of the Systems Framework for Healthy Policy (Commonwealth 2016; and WFPHA 2016):

Governance: public health legislation; policy; strategy; financing; organisation; quality assurance: transparency, accountability, and audit.

Knowledge: surveillance, monitoring, and evaluation; research and evidence; risk and innovation; dissemination and uptake.

Protection: IHR and co-ordination; communicable disease control; emergency preparedness; environmental health; and climate change and sustainability.

Promotion: inequalities; environmental determinants; social and economic determinants; resilience; behaviour and health literacy; life course; and healthy settings.

Prevention: primary prevention: vaccination; secondary prevention: screening; tertiary prevention: rehabilitation, healthcare management, and planning.

People-centred care: primary healthcare; secondary healthcare; tertiary healthcare; and rehabilitation.

Advocacy: leadership and ethics; community engagement and empowerment; communications; and sustainable development.

Capacity: workforce development for public health workers, health workers, and wider workforce; workforce planning: numbers, resources, and infrastructure; standards, curriculum, and accreditation; and capabilities, teaching, and training.

The Systems Framework for Healthy Policy acts as an overarching framework that embeds Essential Public Health Operations within the health system. A further policy resource builds upon the structure of this framework and outlines in detail the role of the health system as an essential component of Global Security (Commonwealth, 2017). This resource includes an outline of the main challenges to global health security and aims to act as a blueprint for assessing and improving the health protection components summarised below. These frameworks and toolkits were created prior to the COVID-19 pandemic and would benefit from further development, ideally at global level, to address future pandemics and health threats.

Key Components for Health Protection Services (Commonwealth, 2017):

International Health Regulation (IHR) and Co-ordination: this includes strategic planning and co-ordination of health protection services including:

- Communicable disease control, emergency preparedness, and environmental health.
- Service modernisation to address emerging challenges and cross-cutting issues, for example, climate change.
- Coordination, implementation, and governance processes established with national and international partners to contribute to global health security including reporting.

Communicable Disease Control

- Local, regional, national, and international co-ordination and advice.
- Development or adaptation of protocols and guidance for high-risk communicable diseases.
- Investigation and management: diagnosis; quality assurance and co-ordination of public health laboratories; active surveillance and monitoring; treatment of cases; and contact tracing and outbreak investigation.
- Control and response: public education and awareness; preventive action, for example, vaccination; training on infection control; isolation and containment.
- Evaluation: applying learning to improve co-ordination, delivery responses, protocols, guidance, and training.

Emergency Preparedness

- Co-ordination, roles, and responsibilities established with other agencies, sectors and at international, national, regional, and local levels.
- Assessment of risks, identification of priorities, and development of risk registers.
- Development of plans for emergency situations such as pandemic influenza; infectious disease outbreaks; natural disasters such as earthquakes; extreme weather events such as floods, fires, heat and cold; other environmental events threatening human health; mass gatherings; deliberate attacks: industrial accidents – chemical, biological, radiological, nuclear, etc.
- Planning for primary prevention; early warning systems; emergency responses; and ensuring business continuity.
- Short and long-term follow-up, including effects of contamination; physical and mental health impacts; and methods of evaluation.
- Testing and revising plans, incorporating lessons into future training and protocols.

Environmental Health: Proactive action to mitigate harm and react to benefits to health from environmental determinants.

- Local, regional, national, and international co-ordination and advice to maximise sanitation, safety, security, and quality.
- Development or adaptation of protocols and guidance to manage public health risks from different environmental hazards (for example, chemical, physical, radiation, and noise) in different scenarios and environmental media (air, soil, water, and food).
- Aspects of the built environment such as home safety and transport-associated injuries.
- Prevention: legislation, use of alternative chemicals, facility build and process, regulation and enforcement, and development control (influence rural/urban planning processes to minimise exposure potential).
- Preparation: multi-agency planning and training, robust notification and alert arrangements, and public warning systems.
- Detection and alert: operator controls, environmental sampling and monitoring, and effective alert systems.
- Response: risk assessment, risk management, and risk communication to break environmental health source-pathway-receptor linkages.
- Recovery: ongoing health assessment and epidemiological follow-up, clean-up, and investigation of the root cause of an incident or problem to prevent recurrence.
- Evaluation: applying learning to improve co-ordination, delivery responses, protocols, guidance, and training.

Climate Change and Sustainability: Assess health impacts and provide advocacy and policy advice on risks to health and strengthen relevant public health functions to support:

- Adaptation planning and strengthening of health resilience.
- Cross-sector sustainability and mitigation planning that benefits health, the economy, and the environment. Including safe roads and green spaces that promote active transport, building design, and reduction of unhealthy food energy, for example, clean cooking stoves.
- Linking environmental health determinants and benefits with health promotion.

Rapid responses by environmental health professionals are often critical in regulating early preventive efforts and in successfully controlling outbreaks to prevent communal spread. However, in many countries environmental health capacity has been substantially underinvested, depleted, and is often invisible (Day, 2021). Renewal and modernisation of the environmental health profession will be key to preventing pandemics and increasingly for our ability to tackle our Planetary Emergency.

The modernisation of public health will need to address the increasing threats from synthetically created pathogens and will need greater attention, control, and governance measures. Following the COVID-19 pandemic a rapid expansion has occurred of high containment laboratories that are capable of producing genetically modified pathogens. It is estimated that there are now over 100 laboratories worldwide that have the capacity to produce highly lethal pathogens that could be released intentionally or unintentionally with devastating effects. Although the purpose of most of these laboratories is to create vaccines for future mutations, prior to 2000, there were over 1,200 laboratory accidental infections resulting in 22 deaths. An estimated 50% of the new laboratories being created are poorly regulated and are developed within countries with low-security measures. Moreover, there is currently an absence of global governance mechanisms to enable consistent safety and regulation measures in place (Field, 2023).

Preventing Pandemics – A Cost-Effective Investment

To prevent future pandemics, there is a clear role for scaling up essential global, regional, national, and community public health functions and operations, including embedding health protection within our health systems. Ideally, the WHO would play a central role in building capacity at all levels as part of delivering its commitments for Universal Health Coverage. A key barrier so far has been the funding mechanism for the WHO, which mainly relies on voluntary contributions from other international organisations, member states, donors, and philanthropic foundations. This constitutes 80% of the WHO funds and dictates where the WHO can spend its money. Most of the voluntary contributions want to see tangible outcomes, mainly related to specific diseases. Very little funding is allocated to strengthening health protection services and essential public health functions or on strengthening health systems. Furthermore, such isolated disease programmes act to undermine national health systems by pulling health workers into the provision of better-paid single-issue services. Funding to health security tends to go towards specialist laboratory services which are not sustainable as part of national health budgets, nor incorporated as part of the national health system. Instead, donors prefer to fly in such international specialists as the proposed 'pandemic fire brigade' at great cost (Gates, 2022).

Unfortunately, this approach tends to further disempower national health systems and capacity and further reinforces disparities of power between rich and poor countries.

In 2021, the WHO DG estimated that only 3% of national health sector budgets is spent on prevention. Although difficult to estimate, the proportion of this spent on health protection services may only represent two-thirds of this, approximately 2% of the total health budget. Even doubling the health protection budget would only require 5% of the total health budget to be allocated to this critical public health function. This is in stark contrast to the global costs of the COVID-19 pandemic that the International Monetary Fund estimates will reach $12.5 trillion by 2024. In 2019 the Global Preparedness Monitoring Board (GPMB) emphasised the need to prepare for the worse, from either naturally occurring pandemics or from intentional release as part of biological terrorism or warfare. Prior to the COVID-19 pandemic, an estimated $1–2 per person per year (a total of $8–16 billion) was calculated by the World Bank and the WHO as needed to ensure adequate pandemic preparedness worldwide. However, given the weaknesses revealed by the COVID-19 pandemic, this figure may need to be higher. Earlier estimates by the GPMB for strengthening animal and human health systems anticipated a return on investment of 10:1 (GPMB, 2019).

The fact remains that the relative cost of preventing pandemics and strengthening public health operations is substantially less than the devastating costs of responding to a pandemic. The World Bank recently estimated that investment in prevention during the pandemic represented only 1% of the total costs of the pandemic. It highlights the importance of investing in pandemic prevention as a global public health good and recommends investing in early prevention. In particular, it advocates the adoption of a 'One Health' approach, which would cost an estimated $10.3–$11.5 billion per year, consisting of veterinary services, farm biosecurity, and afforestation (World Bank, 2022). Economists have estimated investments for One Health approaches to prevent pandemics require an annual $120–$340 million for viral discovery, and $217–$279 million for early detection and control within 31 high-risk countries (Bernstein et al, 2022). Aside from reducing the risk of animal infections spilling over to humans, many of these investments would also be beneficial for climate change.

Effective Prevention Is Wider Than the Health Sector

Considering the spectrum of measures that can be effectively applied to prevent future pandemics, aside from the important role of mainstreaming public health operations into health systems, relevant aspects need to be embedded across other sectors. As the GPMB stressed in 2019, applying the precautionary principle to assessing risks and planning for the worse is at the heart of effectively preventing a pandemic. Aside from the technical operations and functions required to protect our health, a key aspect of preventing pandemics is by ensuring a resilient and healthy population. That the Spanish 'Flu' was so devastating was in part due to a malnourished and stressed population at the end of World War I. With COVID-19, we have seen how those with weaker immune systems have been at higher risk of serious illness, disability, and death. Moreover, weakened immunity creates more opportunities for pathogens to mutate. In essence, we need to see health as a global good and ensure that the health of everyone, everywhere is looked after. To do so requires multi-sector responses to enhance individual, community, national and global resilience, together with the promotion of human, animal, and environmental health and well-being. There is substantial evidence for multi-sector interventions that are cost-effective and bring short and longer-term returns on investment (WHO Europe, 2014). Many of these interventions bring multiple benefits to the environment and the wider community. An integrated response to the promotion of physical and mental health is a key aspect of enhancing resilience in the prevention of pandemics. This requires the promotion of healthy policies that enhance the determinants of health, spanning across the life course, and social, economic, and environmental factors. Increasingly, the role of digital technology and innovation makes this a possibility for all as a common good (P4PPP, 2022).

Recognising health as a Human Right is a fundamental principle for protecting the health of everyone. To achieve this, addressing inequalities in health needs to be done systematically, across communities, countries, and around the world. Regarding health as a global good will become increasingly important in preventing pandemics and other global threats to health. Health security should be part of cross-governmental emergency and contingency planning for national security. Pandemic prevention needs to be incorporated within emergency systems as part of the Sendai Framework for Disaster Risk Reduction. The implications for leadership will be explored further later in the book. Recognising the role of health as an essential component of Global Security is critical and is discussed in the final chapter.

Key Messages

- **Was the COVID-19 Pandemic Preventable?** Yes. The pandemic could have been prevented if there had been better preparedness and swifter action, clearer communication of risks and alerts, greater global coordination with ambitious and strategic leadership, the creation of vaccines as a global good, and robust public health systems in place.
- **Prevention – A Critical Concept:** preventing a pandemic from happening in the first place reduces overall harm to people and the economy; elimination plans are recommended as the first response for future pandemics; the

wider concepts of prevention, from primary to quaternary prevention need to be applied within the context of pandemics.

- **Learn from Success to Prevent Future Pandemics:** an Emergency Framework for Countries and Communities for COVID-19 should be introduced, which builds upon early responses by countries that successfully controlled the pandemic.
- **Essential Public Health Operations:** should be embedded as core components of the health system, to ensure a sustainable and scalable response to pandemics, with modernised health protection and environmental health functions to address our wider global health threats.
- **Preventing Pandemics – A Cost-Effective Investment:** the estimated global costs of the COVID-19 pandemic amounted to $12.5 trillion by 2024; in contrast, pandemic preparedness is estimated to cost $8–$16 billion globally per year. Increased investment is required for preventive services, which currently represent only 3% of the average health sector budget.
- **Effective Prevention is wider than the Health Sector:** pandemics are less likely to occur with healthy humans, animals, and environments. Multi-sector prevention is a cost-effective response with returns on investment and multiple benefits. Pandemic prevention needs to be part of mainstream emergency and security responses. In the future, digital solutions can potentially play a key role in coordination, scale, and speed.

Bibliography

Baker M G et al, (2020) 'Elimination Could be the Optimal Response Strategy for COVID-19 and Other Emerging Pandemic Diseases' *BMJ* 371: m4907.

Bernstein A et al, (2022) 'The Costs and Benefits of Primary Prevention of Zoonotic Pandemics' *Science Advances*, 4th Feb; 8(5). DOI:10.1126/sciadv.abl4183

Commonwealth (2016) 'A Systems Framework for Healthy Policy – Advancing Global Health Security and Sustainable Well-Being for All' Implementation Tool for the 'Global Charter for the Public's Health': www.thecommonwealth-healthhub.net

Commonwealth (2017a) 'The Role of Health in Contributing to Global Security' A policy brief; the Commonwealth Secretariat: www.thecommonwealth-healthhub.net

Commonwealth (2017b) 'The Case for Investing in Health' A policy brief; the Commonwealth Secretariat: www.thecommonwealth-healthhub.net

Commonwealth (2017c) 'Health Protection Policy Toolkit: Health as an Essential Component of Global Security'; 2nd Edition: www.thecommonwealth-healthhub.net

Day C ed, (2021) 'COVID-19: The Global Environmental Health Experience' the Chartered Institute of Environmental Health; Routledge, Focus.

Field M, (2023) 'Despite Risk-Management Gaps, Countries Press Ahead with New Labs That Study Deadly Pathogens' Bulletin of the Atomic Scientists: https://thebulletin.org/2023/01/despite-risk-management-gaps-countries-press-ahead-with-new-labs-that-study-deadly-pathogens/

Gates B, (2022) '*How to Prevent the Next Pandemic*' Penguin.

GPMB (2019) 'A World at Risk - Annual Report on Global Preparedness for Health Emergencies' Global Preparedness Monitoring Board.

IAC (2020) 'COVID-19 Policy Framework for Global, National and Community Responses' The InterAction Council: https://www.interactioncouncil.org/index.php/media-centre/council-former-world-leaders-urges-urgent-global-co-operation-combat-covid-19-and-plan

IPPPR (2021) 'COVID-19: Make It the Last Pandemic' International Panel for Pandemic Preparedness and Response.

Misra M et al, (2022) 'Exit Strategies from Lockdowns Due to COVID-19: A Scoping Review' *BMC Public Health*, Mar 12; 22(1): 488.

Oliu-Barton et al, (2022) 'Elimination Versus Mitigation of SARS-CoV-2 in the Presence of Effective Vaccines' The Lancet, Global Health, Jan 2022; 10(1): E142–E147.

P4PPP (2022) 'Creating Digital Solutions for Pandemics and Global Health Security' https://drive.google.com/file/d/1ig-VTUaHCKCsE4GhXUvoS0og7RK9EwUG/view

P4PPP (2022) 'Creating Digital Futures: Platform for Planet, Place and People, (P4PPP); Progress and Plans 2022-2027' https://sites.google.com/view/p4ppp/resources

Sendai Framework (2015) '*Sendai Framework for Disaster Risk Reduction 2015-2030*' UNDRR.

Wenham C et al, (2022) 'The Futility of the Pandemic Treaty: Caught Between Globalism and Statism' *International Affairs*, May; 98(2): 837–852.

WFPHA (2016) 'A Global Charter for the Public's Health – The Public Health System: Role, Functions, Competencies and Education Requirements' *The European Journal of Public Health*, Mar 8: https://www.wfpha.org/images/PHAA01001_Global-Charter_PROOF_160812_FINAL.pdf

WHO, Europe 2012: 'The European Action Plan and Resolution for Strengthening Public Health Services and Capacity' WHO Europe, 2012, WHO RC 62: www.euro.who.int/publichealth

WHO, Europe 2012: 'Review of Public Health Capacities and Services in the European Region' www.euro.who.int/publichealth

WHO, Europe 2012: 'Preliminary Review of Institutional Models for Delivering Essential Public Health Operations in Europe' www.euro.who.int/publichealth

WHO, Europe 2012: 'Public Health Policy and Legislation Instruments and Tools: An Updated Review and Proposal for Further Research' www.euro.who.int/publichealth

WHO Europe 2014: 'The Case for Investing in Public Health' www.euro.who.int/publichealth

WHO (2018) 'Essential Public Health Functions, Health Systems and Health Security - Developing Conceptual Clarity and a WHO Roadmap for Action' World Health Organization, Geneva.

WHO (2021) 'Building Health Systems Resilience for Universal Health Coverage and Health Security During the COVID-19 Pandemic and Beyond: WHO Position Paper' World Health Organization, Geneva.

World Bank (2022) 'Putting Pandemics Behind Us: Investing in One Health to Reduce Risks of Emerging Infectious Diseases' Washington DC, World Bank.

7 Lessons for Our Planetary Emergency

Our Planetary Emergency – We Cannot Afford to Fail

In many respects, looking back in time, we can be seen to have failed in our attempts to prevent and contain the pandemic at the cost of millions of lives, widening inequalities, human rights abuses, democratic collapse, and to the detriment of achieving the sustainable development goals. However, the COVID-19 pandemic, along with other pandemics, will pale into insignificance in comparison to the threats to the existence of life posed by the Planetary Emergency. Our current and future environmental, biodiversity, and climate crises are described in this book as the Planetary Emergency, which can be seen as a driving force for the majority of other threats to life, including pandemics, migration, conflicts, and wars. The escalating interaction of these reinforcing risks to human existence has been described as a poly-crisis of existential threats to human security (Nurse, 2023) and has been summarised in Chapter 3.

Current evidence reveals that a number of planetary tipping points are being exceeded. Once certain critical temperatures have been reached, there is a danger that the Earth's natural cooling mechanisms will no longer be able to maintain the temperatures compatible with human life. The ice caps have started to melt at increasing speed, along with the warming of permafrost regions that are releasing methane – which in turn creates further warming. This is described as a positive feedback loop, whereby each of the Earth's cooling systems can reinforce each other in a process that can rapidly escalate further global warming. Unlike the false reassurance conveyed by the 2022 IPCC report, of 'temporary overshoots' this process may not be easy to reverse. Examining the history of the Earth, this process normally takes millennia to reverse, by which time human civilisation as well as much of the life on this Earth will be long gone.

The next few years may be described in medical terms as the 'Golden Hour' of Planet Earth: the first hour after a life-threatening injury when the treatment is critical to the patient's survival. With multi-system failures, the Earth's chance of survival depends upon our rapidly moving it into intensive care (IAC, 2019). Of course, the planet itself will survive, but what is at risk

DOI: 10.1201/9781003181088-7

is the Earth's 'biosphere', which allows humans and the majority of other forms of life to exist (Kump et al, 2016). What is at stake is our ability to save a liveable planet. Rather than a golden hour, we probably have a few golden years in which to rapidly cool the Earth, stabilise, and potentially reverse the system's tipping points. Some authors consider that as a relatively ageing and frail planet, the Earth's systems are less resilient to rapid changes (Lovelock, 2019). This could mean that if it continues to experience the multiple shocks that are occurring within the context of the current poly-crisis, the decline in its cooling systems could accelerate further. The worst-case scenario could be the creation of a super-hot planet like Venus, lacking water and oxygen, with no biosphere for life.

This is a critical time for our very survival. We cannot afford to fail in preventing a catastrophic future for humanity and much of life on Earth. Our ability to apply lessons from the pandemic will be seen as a trial run for our ability to turn around the Planetary Emergency. However, Doctors can now revive a critical patient, even at death's door, bringing them back to life and enabling a healthy recovery. There is still hope, but it will depend upon our capability to stabilise our ailing planet and set it on track for a healthy recovery where all can flourish.

Key Lessons from the Pandemic for our Planetary Emergency

The pandemic had a relatively slow start which was mostly ignored or denied; however, it rapidly escalated and overwhelmed us. Although our Planetary Emergency is running on a different timeframe of years and decades rather than days and months, the process of exponential escalation is similar. The critical time where the most difference can be made to prevent pandemics is early on. With the Planetary Emergency, we are like frogs in a pan that is gradually heating. Some of us are even enjoying the extra warmth, but, if we do not act soon, the situation will become too hot for us to escape. This section revisits the key points for how we failed, and what we could have done to prevent the pandemic in order to draw out learning for our Planetary Emergency.

The points below apply the lessons from how we failed to prevent the pandemic to the Planetary Emergency.

- **Ignored Risks:** we know that the Planetary Emergency is a very high risk and impact series of events; risks are being denied by such terms as 'temporary overshoot'.
- **Underinvested:** we are substantially under-investing in solutions to rapidly decarbonise our energy sources and secure essential biospheres, at national, regional, and global levels – so neglecting our insurance system for preventing the Planetary Emergency.

- **Prepared for the Wrong Thing:** we have a narrow risk perspective on the Planetary Emergency, focusing largely on 1–2°C rather than preparing for and preventing worst-case scenarios.
- **Failed to act at a Critical Stage:** many political leaders are ignoring and denying early alerts and warning signs as we exceed tipping points and lose valuable time.
- **Reaction versus Prevention:** globally our projected emissions put us on a trajectory of escalating temperatures, yet we largely continue to react to damages and aim to reduce its impact, rather than focusing on early prevention. This is analogous to reacting to the pandemic by relying on hospital treatment and allowing people to die.
- **Fragmented Responses:** around the world the emphasis has been on building consensus with commitments that are rarely fulfilled, and often serve to shift accountability elsewhere.
- **Lack of Political Leadership:** we lack substantial political commitment for an international strategic and coordinated response to match the scale of response required to address our Planetary Emergency.
- **National versus Global Responses:** the rise of populism has encouraged some politicians to act with self-interest and widen inequalities; allowing fossil fuel companies (and their profits) to influence decisions, makes it increasingly difficult to mount a global response.
- **Becoming Overwhelmed:** many people feel hopeless about the future; however, we are still in the 'Golden Years' where there is time to act at speed and scale.

Critical Areas for the Planetary Emergency – Lessons from the Pandemic

The below points outline key areas that could have acted to prevent the pandemic and if applied to the Planetary Emergency could have the potential to turn around our projected global catastrophe. The next section considers each area further in turn.

- **Digital Platforms for Global Coordination and Strategic Action:** the U.N. system has the ability to facilitate the mobilisation of political commitment and coordinate strategic action to address the Planetary Emergency. This will require strengthening of the international architecture which could be enabled through digital platforms.
- **Prevention, Preparedness, and Risk Reduction:** we could invest in robust and flexible community, national, regional, and international plans that built upon the Sendai Framework with an all-hazards multi-sector approach. This could include a strong emphasis on resilience, surveillance, detection, early warning systems, and responses, with a drive for

prevention and early interventions. The communication of risks of exceeding critical temperatures and tipping point thresholds need to be clearly communicated for politicians and policymakers.

- **An Emergency Response to the Determinants of Life on Earth:** including air, water, food, land, and a healthy biosphere with a liveable temperature, need to be stabilised rapidly with emergency responses and be regarded as global goods for human security.
- **Create a Health System for Our Planet Earth:** the development of an emergency response for the Earth and the protection of our Planet's Health requires bringing together existing disciplines and professional bodies with a common agenda of securing a healthy planet for all.

Digital Platforms for Global Coordination and Strategic Action

Innovation and digital technology already have the potential to enable the transformation needed to enhance global coordination and strategic actions. Drawing on lessons from the pandemic, we already have significant knowledge and systems created by the digital technology within our reach. These are described in Figure 7.1.

This diagram adapts material from the report 'Creating Digital Solutions for Pandemics and Global Health Security' by the Platform for Planet, Place, and People (P4PPP, 2022), an initiative developed by the Commonwealth Centre for Digital Health, with the vision of transforming future health systems as a common good for all. It builds upon the core public health operations embedded within the Systems Framework for Healthy Policy (Commonwealth, 2016) and the Health Protection Policy Toolkit (Commonwealth, 2017) both

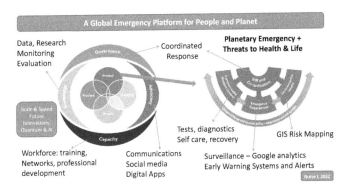

Figure 7.1 Lessons from the Pandemic – Digital Solutions for People and Planet

of which were outlined in the previous chapter. Examples of digital technologies that already exist for Global Health Security, including our Planetary Emergency can be found on the Digital Platform for Planet, Place, and People (P4PPP, 2022).

These studies include tools for managing and sharing knowledge, including data, evaluation, monitoring, and research. They have been applied to health protection functions with Geographical Information Systems (GIS) risk mapping, surveillance, and early warning systems for climate change. Social media and digital apps already exist to facilitate mass communication and can be further developed to garner community responses. Online education, training, and professional programmes have been in operation for over a decade, with the flexibility to create new educational programmes rapidly through Massive Open Online Courses (MOOCs). The application of artificial intelligence also has the potential to create complex analyses for critical thresholds and trigger responses to address the Earth's interacting systems. In the near future, it is anticipated that quantum computing will transform the way the world functions, operating at super speed and with the ability to rapidly analyse complex scenarios. An increasingly important role of digital platforms will be their ability to coordinate strategic global responses rapidly.

Prevention, Preparedness, and Risk Reduction

Even the best-case scenarios for rises in temperature place our future in a catastrophic situation. If we were to achieve all the unconditional, nationally determined contributions and implement the net zero targets, we would only be on track to reach an estimated 1.6–1.9°C by 2100. In reality, the U.N. Environment Programme's Emissions Gap Report for 2022 estimated that, on our current policy trajectory, we are most likely to reach 2.8°C by the end of this century (UNEP, 2022). Furthermore, these calculations have not fully factored in cascading rises in temperature due to exceeding tipping points. Based upon current policy trajectories, global temperatures are likely to exceed 3°C and to continue rising in the following century, potentially reaching up to 10°C.

Of particular concern is our interpretation and relative denial of risks. We are currently on track to reach temperatures that equate to mass extinction, but many climate policy reports present false reassurances. For example, even with the best-case scenario, we will not be able to maintain temperatures below 1.5°C. On the IPPC 2022 best-case scenario, there is a 90% chance of reaching temperatures of 1.6–1.9°C by 2100. Furthermore, this estimate includes having a 'temporary overshoot' peaking at between 1.9 and 2.1°C during this century. The concept of temporary overshoot provides a false sense of optimism and masks the substantial risks that we face. Unfortunately, policymakers who do not have a full understanding of scientific principles tend to present findings that are acceptable to their political leaders.

A comprehensive risk analysis which includes the risks from multiple sources such as cascading tipping points and the application of the precautionary principle is required urgently. In reality, at an increase of just 1.1°C global surface temperature, we are already experiencing the start of cascading tipping points which will continue to drive up temperatures further. To avert runaway, climate change with the creation of an unliveable hothouse Earth requires a major shift in global responses (IAC, 2019). Learning from the pandemic, the application of the principles of early prevention to reduce harm and stop the occurrence of catastrophic outcomes will be key. Drawing upon learning from the pandemic, the application of public health concepts of prevention can be applied to our planetary emergency and are described below:

- **Primary Prevention:** whereby the onset of the threat or hazard is prevented from occurring – this requires risk assessment and enhanced resilience.
- **Secondary Prevention:** early detection with early intervention is applied to halt and reverse the progression of the hazard – this is often seen as risk reduction with adaption and early warning systems, including those for tipping point thresholds.
- **Tertiary Prevention:** to make an established problem less severe in order to improve outcomes – this relates to the concepts of treatments and mitigation.
- **Quaternary Prevention:** involves rehabilitation and recovery and relates to the concept of Building Back Better, a strategy aimed at reducing the risks in the wake of future disasters and shocks.

An Emergency Response to the Determinants of Life on Earth

For most of us, a few degrees do not sound like much to worry about and may even seem welcome on a cold winter day. However, a mere 3–4° temperature rise is enough to kill a human being. Moreover, we are already moving into unknown territory, with human civilisation having existed between a comfortable and stable temperature range of −1 to +1°C over the last 800,000 years (IAC, 2019). In 2023, with just a rise of 1.1°C rise, we are already experiencing substantial changes to the climate and environment. The temperature chart below summarises the key impacts as global temperatures rise:

Predicted Risks from the Earth's Temperature Chart

- **One Degree Celsius** = Increased storms and wildfires; with risk of 3–14% extinction of species at 1.5°C
- **Two Degrees Celsius** = Disappearance of Arctic sea ice, widespread droughts; 3–18% of species risk extinction
- **Three Degrees Celsius** = Global food crisis and Amazon Rainforest collapse; 3–29% of species risk extinction
- **Four Degrees Celsius** = China and India largely uninhabitable; 3–39% of species risk extinction
- **Five Degrees Celsius** = Mass extinctions occur; 3–48% of species risk extinction
- **Six Degrees Celsius** = Possible human extinction

(Adapted from Lynas, 2020 and IPCC, 2022)

There are certain critical temperatures that will make the Earth unliveable. Above 15°C, the surface of the sea becomes less able to support life, which is why the waters are clear in hot places. Above 47°C without protection, humans and many other animals are unable to survive metabolically (Lovelock, 2019). Already in 2022, the world experienced more days with extreme temperatures exceeding 47°C than ever before and this will continue to increase. We are moving from a time of stable temperatures and climatic conditions to an era of rapidly escalating temperatures. In the context of geological epochs, this is described as the Anthropocene – a new era dominated by human activity that is creating an escalation in global temperatures (Lewis and Maslin, 2018).

Although perceived as controversial by some, in the 1970s, James Lovelock recognised that the Earth's systems operated in a similar way to a living organism. With Lynn Margulis, he named this concept the 'Gaia Hypothesis' after the Greek Goddess of Earth. Parallels are made with the way living organisms self-regulate complex and interacting systems in order to create and maintain conditions favourable to life (Boston et al, 2008). This theory has since been developed and grown into a scientific discipline described as 'Earth Systems' (Kump et al, 2016). Since the initial concept of the Gaia Hypothesis was published, Lovelock has gone on to describe how the Earth's systems are analogous to that of the health, physiology, and metabolism seen within animals (Lovelock, 2000).

Although, not precisely the same, there are substantial parallels between how Earth Systems operate with that of life systems observed within animals. This is not surprising, given that all life has evolved from the Earth over time, and the planet can be seen as our common ancestor, as well as our home. If we consider Planet Earth as a living system, it is possible to see that its health is in a critical state (IAC, 2019). Rather than the slow and largely unsubstantial actions that have been taken so far, we should recognise the necessity to take emergency action. This will need to involve more than achieving net zero targets, as the harm inflicted upon the Earth's vital systems is far more substantial than that reflected by carbon emissions alone. We have only a critical few years, in which to slow down and hopefully reverse what can be seen as multi-system organ failure, resulting in cascading changes to our Earth's climate systems, with major temperature rises and mass extinctions.

Picking up the analogy of the 'Golden Hour' again, it is vital that such 'Golden Years' as remain before us should be used wisely. To secure the survival of future generations, we need to generate an emergency response in order to stabilise the Earth's health system. In an emergency situation in animals, vital life signs are determined by the ABC of Airways, Breathing, and Circulation – equivalent to Earth's Air and Water systems. In intensive care, the functions of the major organs need to be maintained and sustained to prevent multi-system failure. In the analogy, this equates to Food, while Land represents the skin with the final stages of systemic shock observed just before death. Air, Water, Food, and Land (or a place to live) can be seen as the essential determinants for all life forms. Without them, we cannot exist. The emergency responses to ensure the Vital Determinants of Life (P4PPP, 2023) are outlined below. These build upon existing evidence including that from the Drawdown project, the Lancet EAT Commission, Nature-Based Solutions, Planetary Boundary's, and NASA's vital statistics for the Earth.

Emergency Responses to Ensure the Vital Determinants of Life (P4PPP, 2023)

Temperature: 1.1°C increase since 1880
Air:

- **Indicators:** carbon dioxide – 420 ppm and other warming gases.
- **Energy:** rapid investment and scaling up of renewable energy.
- **Transport:** major transition of transport systems based upon renewable energy and active transport (walking and cycling).
- **Clean Air:** carbon sequestration to rapidly reduce carbon emissions.

Water:

- **Indicators:** ocean acidity; ocean warming; loss of ice sheets; and sea level rise.
- **Oceans:** enhance the Oceans' health by recovering planetary homeostasis (temperature, acidity, toxins, and plastics).

- **Land Water:** advance nature-based solutions including maintaining and increasing swamps, peat bogs, flood planes, and aquifers.

Food:

- **Indicators:** energy intensity of food systems; environmental toxins.
- **Anabolic:** scale up sustainable 'Healthy Planetary Food Systems' that enable a nutritious and healthy planet.
- **Catabolic:** reduce excess consumption and food waste, improve storage, clean cooking, recycle waste, and refrigeration.
- **Toxins:** reduce environmental toxins and restore contaminated environments.

Land:

- **Indicators**: desertification; forestation; and soil quality and acidity.
- **Environment:** restore diverse habitats with nature-based solutions; reverse desertification and enhance reforestation.
- **Earth:** enhance soil health and carbon uptake.
- **Albedo:** design environments to maximise reflection and aid cooling with white surfaces.

Create a Health System for Our Planet Earth

To scale up the emergency responses to ensure that the vital determinants for our Planets' life systems are secured requires a coordinated infrastructure and services. This could take the form of a health system for Planet Earth. The main determinants of life together with the operations required for an emergency response to secure a healthy planet for all are described in the graphic table below. These include governance and guardianship, including legislation, policy, strategic responses, leadership, resources, and accountability mechanisms. Security includes preventive measures and emergency interventions to stabilise our Planet's Health, including the symptoms of storms, floods, droughts, and fires. These responses are informed by the application of information and knowledge, including digital technology, to create an emergency response to ensure our global security. Once the emergency situation has been stabilised, a longer-term recovery plan is required to enable the planet to regain its health and resilience. Providing a sense of hope is a key aspect of the healing process, and empowering young people and communities to create a liveable future and flourishing planet for all will also play a critical role (Hickman et al, 2021).

These operations along with the main determinants of life are captured within the framework below which describes a 'Health System for our Planet Earth'. This draws upon the concept described as a Universal Health Systems for Planet, Place and People in the Manifesto to Secure a Healthy Planet for All (IAC, 2019) which has been further advanced by the Digital Platform for Planet Place and People (P4PPP).

Universal Health Systems for Planet, Place and People (IAC, 2019)

1 **Governance:** planetary health guardianship and legislation; science-based policy and strategy; cyclical investment; and planetary health index.

2 **Knowledge:** surveillance, monitoring, and evaluation; research and evidence; risk and innovation; and digital systems and dissemination.

3 **Protection:** planetary health – risks and response; International Health Regulations and Sendai Framework; communicable disease control; emergency preparedness; environmental health; and climate change and sustainability.

4 **Promotion:** intergenerational inequalities; AIR-WATER-LAND-FOOD systems; co-benefits and sustainable development; ecological health literacy; life-course resilience; and healthy eco-settings.

5 **Prevention:** primary prevention: vaccination; secondary prevention: screening; efficient healthcare management, waste, and recycling.

6 **People:** primary health care (ecological community officers; maternal and child health); secondary and tertiary health and social care and recovery.

7 **Advocacy:** leadership and ethics; planetary health community guardians; green connected communities; and multi-media networks.

8 **Capacity:** life-course education, workforce development; workforce planning: numbers, resources, infrastructure; standards, curriculum, accreditation; and capabilities, teaching, and training (Figure 7.2).

In creating a health system for Planet Earth, we can draw upon lessons from the pandemic, including emergency care and treatment, together with learning how to build sustainable human health systems. This could include the application of preventive measures and public health operations as well as disaster risk reduction responses from the Sendai Framework. The professional and practitioner roles of the environmental health community have

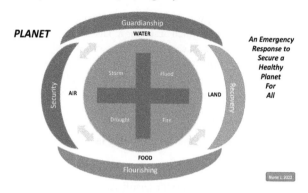

Figure 7.2 A Health System for Our Planet Earth (P4PPP)

many substantial transferable skills that could be applied to the creation of a healthy planet. The concept of 'One Health' builds upon the discipline of environmental health, though it is primarily led by the veterinary profession, which, in order to secure human health, has largely focused upon the health of animals. The recently developed field of 'Planetary Health' has so far mainly focused upon climate and environmental health research and their impacts upon humanity. Yet, as it evolves there is scope within this emerging field to incorporate the health of the planet. There are possibilities of modernising existing training and professional programmes and of creating a new trans-disciplinary field that focuses primarily on the health of Planet Earth. This could apply knowledge, systems, and professional development from existing programmes. This concept is described further in the next chapters.

Key Messages

- **Our Planetary Emergency – We Cannot Afford to Fail:** current policies place us on a potential trajectory for 3°C by 2100, which risks global temperatures escalating with the creation of a hothouse Earth and unliveable world.
- **Applying Lessons from the Pandemic:** there are parallels with the pandemic response, including a lack of preparedness and failure to act at critical stages; we need greater global leadership with coordinated strategic responses.
- **Digital Platforms for Global Coordination and Strategic Action:** existing digital technology has the potential to enhance risk analysis and solutions, surveillance, early alerts, scale-up capacity, and communicate and coordinate strategic responses globally.

- **Prevention, Preparedness, and Risk Reduction:** we are not matching action with the size and scale of the risks, and need to apply the precautionary principle to worst-case scenarios and invest in a range of prevention measures.
- **An Emergency Response for the Determinants of Life on Earth:** the size and scale of our planetary emergency requires an urgent emergency response to address the critical determinants of the Earth's life systems including air, water, food, and land.
- **Create A Health System for our Planet Earth:** we can create a transdisciplinary approach to securing our Earth's health by applying knowledge and operational systems from environmental health and other related approaches including Public Health, the Sendai Framework, One Health, and Planetary Health.

Bibliography

Boston P J, (2008) 'Gaia Hypothesis' Encyclopedia of Ecology: https://www.sciencedirect.com/topics/earth-and-planetary-sciences/gaia-hypothesis

Club of Rome (2019 and 2020) 'The Planetary Emergency Plan and the Planetary Emergency 2.0'; By The Club of Rome, in partnership with Potsdam Institute for Climate Impact Research: https://www.clubofrome.org/publication/the-planetary-emergency-plan/

EAT – Lancet Commission Summary Report (2019) 'Food in the Anthropocene: The EAT-Lancet Commission on Healthy Diets from Sustainable Food Systems' (Walter Willett et al.): https://eatforum.org/eat-lancet-commission/eat-lancetcommission-summary-report/

Figueres C, Schellnhuber H J, Whiteman G, Rockstrom J, Hobley A and Rahmstorf S, (2017) 'Three Years to Safeguard our Climate' *Nature*, June 29; 546: 593–595. www.nature.com/news/three-years-to-safeguard-ourclimate-1.22201

Friedman T L, (2009) '*Hot Flat and Crowded – Why the World Needs a Green Revolution and How We Can Renew our Global Future*' Penguin.

Hawken P ed, (2017) 'Drawdown: The Most Comprehensive Plan Ever Proposed to Reverse Global Warming' Paul Hawken (Ed), Penguin: www.drawdown.org

Hickman C et al, (2021) 'Climate Anxiety in Children and Young People and Their Beliefs About Government Responses to Climate Change: A Global Survey' *The Lancet, Planetary Health* 5(12): E863–E873.

IAC (2019). 'Manifesto to Secure a Healthy Planet for All – A Call for Emergency Action' The InterAction Council: https://www.interactioncouncil.org/publications/manifesto-secure-healthy-planet-all-call-emergency-action

IPCC (2022) 'IPCC Sixth Assessment Report' Policy Summary: https://www.ipcc.ch/report/ar6/wg2/

Kemp L et al, (2022) 'Climate Endgame: Exploring Catastrophic Climate Change Scenarios' *Proceedings of the National Academy of Sciences/PNAS*, Aug 1; 119: 34.

Kump L R et al, (2016) '*The Earth System*' Pearson.

Lawrence M, Janzwood S and Homer-Dixon T, (2022) 'What Is a Global Polycrisis? And How Is It Different from a Systemic Risk?' Version 2, 2022- 4; Cascade Institute: https://cascadeinstitute.org/technical-paper/what-is-a-global-polycrisis/

Lawrence M M, (2022) '"Polycrisis" may be a buzzword, but it could help us tackle the world's woes' The Conversation: https://theconversation.com/polycrisis-may-be-a-buzzword-but-it-could-help-us-tackle-the-worlds-woes-195280

Lewis S L and Maslin M A, (2018) '*The Human Planet – How we created the Anthropocene*' Pelican Books.

Lovelock J, (2000) '*GAIA – The Practical Science of Planetary Medicine*' Gaia Books Ltd.

Lovelock J, (2019) '*Novacene - The Coming Age of Hyperintelligence*' Allen Lane, Penguin.

Lueddeke G R, (2019) '*Survival: One Health, One Planet, One Future*' Routledge: www.routledge.com/Survival-One-Health-One-Planet-OneFuture/Lueddeke/p/book/9781138334953517

Lynas M, (2020) '*Our Final Warning – Six Degrees of Climate Emergency*' 4th Estate, Harper Collins.

NASA Earth's vital statistics: https://climate.nasa.gov/earth-now/#/

Nature Based Solutions www.naturebasedsolutionsinitiative.org

Nurse J, Moore M, Castro A, Dorey S and Laaser U, (2016) 'A Systems Framework for Healthy Policy – Advancing Global Health Security and Sustainable Well-Being for All' Implementation Tool for the 'Global Charter for the Public's Health' The Commonwealth Secretariat, London, UK: www.thecommonwealth-healthhub.net

Nurse J, (2023) '*Human Security and Existential Threats – A Governance Framework for Planet, Peace, People and Prosperity*' Cadmus, World Academy of Art and Science.

Nurse J, Basher D, Bone A and Bird W, (2010) "An Ecological Approach to Promoting Population Mental Health and Well-being – A Response to the Challenge of Climate Change" *Perspectives in Public Health*, January; 130(1): 27–33.

P4PPP (2022) 'Creating Digital Solutions for Pandemics and Global Health Security' Platform for Planet Place and People: https://drive.google.com/file/d/1ig-VTUaHCKCsE4GhXUvoS0og7RK9EwUG/view

P4PPP (2023) '*Digital Solutions for Our Planetary Emergency – Creating Common Goods for Global Security*' Platform for Planet Place and People (P4PPP); TBP.

Sandifer Q, Dorey S, Nnoaham K, Shankar G, Watson C, Eze E, Brunt H, Dukes G, Battersby S, Archer P, Gilhooly D, Singh A, Dissanayake V, Wyn-Owen J, Aylward M, McDonald B, Nunn R and Nurse J (2017) '*Health Protection Policy Toolkit: Health as an Essential Component of Global Security*' 2nd Edition; Public Health Wales and the Commonwealth Secretariat: www.thecommonwealth-healthhub.net

Seltenrich N, (2018) 'Down to Earth: The Emerging Field of Planetary Health' *Environmental Health Perspectives* 126(7); doi.org/10.1289/EHP2374

Sendai Framework for Disaster Risk Reduction 2015-2030: www.unisdr.org/we/coordinate/sendai-framework

Spratt and Dunlop (2022) 'Climate Dominoes – Tipping Point Risks for Critical Climate Systems?' BreakThrough: https://www.breakthroughonline.org.au/climatedominoes

Stockholm Resilience Centre (2015) 'The Nine Planetary Boundaries' www.stockholmresilience.org/research/planetary-boundaries/planetary-boundaries/about-the-research/the-nine-planetaryboundaries.html

Steffen W, Richardson K, Rockström J et al, (2015) 'Sustainability. Planetary Boundaries: Guiding Human Development on a Changing Planet' *Science* 347: 1259855.

Stockholm Resilience Centre (2018) 'Hothouse Earth Scenario' www. stockholmresilience.org/research/research-news/2018-08-06-planet-at-risk-of-heading-towards-hothouse-earth-state.html

Steffen W et al, (2018) 'Trajectories of the Earth System in the Anthropocene' *PNAS,* August 14; 115(33): 8252–8259. https://doi. org/10.1073/pnas.181014111.5 www. pnas.org/content/115/33/8252

UNEP, (2022) 'Emissions Gap Report 2022' https://www.unep.org/resources/emissions-gap-report-2022

Whitmee S, Haines A, Beyrer C et al, (2015) 'Safeguarding Human Health in the Anthropocene Epoch: Report of The Rockefeller Foundation-Lancet Commission on Planetary Health' *Lancet* 386: 1973–2028.

WHO (2013) 'Protecting Health from Climate Change – A Seven Country Initiative' http://www.euro.who.int/__data/assets/pdf_file/0019/215524/PROTECTING-HEALTH-FROM-CLIMATE-CHANGE-A-seven-country-initiative.pdf?ua=1

8 Transforming Leadership to Secure our Future Well-Being

Transforming Leadership for Complexity and the Poly-Crisis

Our world is becoming increasingly complex with multiple global challenges that threaten our very existence (Nurse, 2023). The pandemic has revealed fundamental weaknesses in our collective ability to successfully address such challenges. There were significant mismatches in the skills required to deal with such an emergency as the COVID-19 pandemic by many of our leaders. They will need to develop a different and wider skill set if they are to navigate the way through multiple and complex threats and challenges. The concept of a poly-crisis describes these multiple and interacting challenges which often reinforce each other. These were outlined earlier in this book, including the main threats to human health, life, and existence, ranging from pandemics to our planetary emergency, as well as conflicts and wars, and potential risks from technological advances.

In recognition of these increasing threats to human survival, Yehezkel Dror describes our current leadership styles as obsolete (Dror, 2017). He considers that, since our leaders play a pivotal role in global security, they need to learn and adapt rapidly if humanity's future existence is to be secured. To achieve this, leaders need to play an active role in ensuring human and global security, which Dror describes as 'Homo Sapiens Governors'. This entails being able to avoid fatal dangers inherent to the human condition, including reducing behaviour such as recklessness. For example, earlier in this book we saw the damaging impacts that resulted from an over emphasis on dominance-based leadership which tends to be driven by strong egos motivated by power. Containing dangerous risks and preventing threats to humanity requires collective governance, which is described in the last chapter. Qualities that can be cultivated at an individual level include a global perspective and strategic longer-term time frames that can be combined with common ethical values focused on human security. A fundamental transformation in the way that leaders lead is required in order to ensure that we are collectively able to navigate the multiple threats to human existence.

DOI: 10.1201/9781003181088-8

This book has identified a number of key areas where many of our leaders failed in their response to the pandemic, as well as behaviours that created successful responses. What has been learned from this is consolidated in the next sections which outline key skill sets required by leaders in order to deal with our multiple challenges and secure the well-being of future generations. The first section revisits the emotional responses to the pandemic and considers the balance of leadership skills required for dealing with emergencies under the themes of the art and science of leadership. Next, an ecological framework is presented that describes the range of leadership styles required to address complex challenges. The last section outlines how to create and train courageous and wise leaders, and the last chapter focuses upon governance and recommendations.

Balancing the Art and Science of Leadership for Existential Threats

Many political and policy leaders tend to have a background in the arts, economics, business, or law, which generally does not adequately equip them with the scientific skills necessary to appreciate many of our complex challenges. During the pandemic, we saw how most people, including our leaders, were drawn into a reinforcing psychological response to the threats to life described in Figure 8.1 under the headings of Threats, Risks, Denial, Panic, Populism and Heroism. Leaders need to avoid being drawn into such a cycle of fear in order to be able to interpret risks and calmly steer their population through a crisis (Gardner, 2009). To be able to do so requires awareness of this pattern of reactions during an emergency, combined with the balanced and robust skill sets described under the themes of the science and art of leadership.

The Science of Leadership: an appreciation of scientific principles and the ability to be able to interpret scientific data are key skills for dealing with

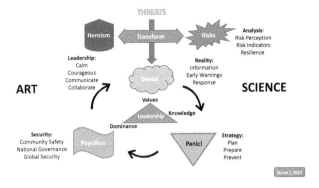

Figure 8.1 The Science and Art of Leadership for Existential Threats

complex challenges and emergencies. Possessing a core scientific skill set enables a greater ability to perceive risks and interpret fact from fiction, thus avoiding political decisions based upon distorted views and misinformation (Rosling et al, 2018). Ideally, risk management and risk governance should become key features in the development of political leaders. Possessing a greater understanding of the nature of and reactions to risks allows for the possibility of preventing disasters from occurring, and for developing comprehensive preparedness plans and processes for if and when they occur (Gardner, 2009). During a crisis, having a scientific skill set allows leaders to be able to actively engage with and scrutinise key evidence-based decisions which are often required in complex emergencies. Relying entirely upon experts and advisors depends upon how well they have been chosen for the tasks required. Many pandemic scientific and medical advisors tended to come from a narrow academic background. Although they were expert researchers within their fields, they were not always competent in responding to an emergency, delivering services, communicating with the public, or influencing multi-sector responses.

Dealing with emergencies requires the application of scientific skills to create effective strategies to underpin prevention, preparedness, and response, together with action plans, the monitoring of processes, and financial accountability (Adair, 2002). Leaders need not be scientists themselves, but they need to have the ability to understand, interpret, and question scientific responses to ensure that good evidence-based decisions are made. The ability to identify what we know, what we don't know, and what is made up will become an increasingly important factor in making sound and balanced decisions for political leaders in the post-truth world (Harari, 2018). Leaders also need to ensure that the right skill sets for senior advisory roles are in place, including successfully leading on creating preventative and emergency systems within complex situations. In emergencies, the adoption of transformational leadership styles is vital in order to consult experts, make collaborative and transparent decisions, and have the ability to rapidly adapt to constant change and uncertainty (Desyatnikov, 2020).

The Art of Leadership: includes the ability to motivate, inspire, influence, coordinate staff, organisations, and populations. The ability to communicate values with a narrative that a wide audience can easily understand is a key part of the art of leadership (Westen, 2007). During the pandemic, although many leaders could be seen to be skilled in aspects of the art of leadership, some leaders utilised this to gain personal power based upon populist narratives. This demonstrates that a balance of skills is required including scientific knowledge and ability, to ensure that the narrative has substance and drives action that protects the whole population. When there is an absence of evidence, communicating values and principles become increasingly important to guide strategic decision-making (Cleary, 1990). The art of leadership includes self-awareness, social and emotional intelligence, as well as an understanding of group dynamics and the ability to be resilient during a crisis (Goleman, 2002). These form the basis of soft leadership skills, including influencing, diplomacy, and the ability to coordinate and collaborate.

The art of leadership also creates the foundation for heroic leadership – as long as it is based upon ethical values and has a strategic direction that has the interests of the whole population at heart. Many of the skill sets described as the art of leadership have also been described under the concept of transformational leadership (HBR, 2011). These include such skills as the ability to act with integrity, build trust and capacity in others and create a collaborative culture based upon a sense of purpose that enables diverse and innovative solutions (Newton et al, 2023). During a crisis, 'heroic leaders' have the ability to be courageous and stay calm in order to oversee coordination and communication during the emergency. To be effective heroic leadership needs to be informed by knowledge and based upon strong values to ensure everybody's security. Balancing the art and science of leadership engenders the ability to see the whole picture, untangle complexity and create innovative solutions. Furthermore, it protects against group-think. The next section expands further on the importance of balancing our intrinsic evolutionary leadership styles expressed as values, knowledge, and dominance-based patterns.

An Ecological Leadership Framework for Complex Global Challenges

With the increasing frequency of emergencies and catastrophic disasters, the ability to apply dynamic and balanced leadership responses to crises will become increasingly important. Drawing on what has been learned from this pandemic, the framework for 'Ecological Leadership for Complex Challenges' is illustrated below. This draws upon ecological principles to apply evolutionary learning to re-orientate existing leadership approaches towards addressing our multiple and complex global challenges. The central triangle and the text boxes describe a dynamic response to apply the best of our intrinsic leadership qualities: values, knowledge, and dominance patterns in response to emergencies and complex challenges, of which key aspects and interactions are summarised below.

- **Values** – The Heart of Leadership
- **Knowledge** – Dynamic Skills for People and Planet
- **Dominance** – Coordination and Governance for Emergency Leadership

The inverted triangle emphasises those aspects that enable balanced and positive leadership styles that are reinforced through governance, transformation, and sustainability (Figure 8.2).

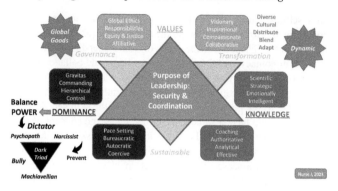

Figure 8.2 An Ecological Leadership Framework for Complex Global Challenges

From the perspective of the planetary emergency, a focus on decision-making based upon sustainable values informed by evidence, coordinated and delivered at pace, will be essential to secure the well-being of future generations. Strengthening transformational leadership skills can enable dynamic and flexible responses that apply a range of balanced and appropriate leadership styles to emergency situations. Building upon this, the concept of Quantum Leadership has recently emerged, based upon principles that inform a vision and purpose, compassion and inclusion, and humility and self-awareness. These combine with knowledge-based skills for independent and creative thinking with the ability to reframe issues and to see the whole picture (Zohar, 2021).

During the pandemic, the ability to ensure a balance between values and knowledge whilst moderating dominance leadership styles enabled effective responses. This balanced style of leadership can be described as transformational or dynamic in nature (Lowder, 2007). It draws upon the best leadership qualities that are applied to a rapidly moving crisis or complex challenge, whilst minimising the negative aspects of each leadership style. For example, a degree of dominant-style behaviour is beneficial to create a sense of security and to enable rapid command-and-control decisions that direct rapid and effective delivery of services. However, the negative aspects of the 'dark triad' traits that came to the fore during the pandemic were characterised by an over-expression of dominant leadership styles that need to be prevented by strong checks and balances. Screening for negative traits early on in leadership selection processes could play an important part in reducing the dangers inherent in the dark triad traits. Actively promoting positive leadership traits for those aspiring to, or holding leadership positions is an important aspect of creating leaders able to deal with increasingly complex challenges. The characteristics of valuing the worth and dignity of each individual (Humanism), not treating people as a means to an end but as an end in their own right (Kantianism), and believing in the fundamental goodness of humanity (Faith in Humanity), have been described as the three values exhibited in the light triad traits of leaders (Kaufman et al, 2019).

We saw in the pandemic how divisive values based upon selfishness and the superiority of one group over another generated populism. Increased nationalism reduced the ability to garner support for the kind of global multi-lateral response which could have brought an effective end to the pandemic. In contrast, a globally recognised set of ethical values based upon a balance of human rights and responsibilities (IAC, 1997) has the potential to act as a tool for collaborative decision-making. It can also provide a strong moral compass for leaders, especially when dealing with chaos, complexity, and uncertainty. Moreover, ethical values can inspire compassion and create a vision of a fair, just, inclusive, and caring world. Transforming our global values could act as a lever to re-orientate financial investments towards the common goods that we all rely on, such as health, the environment, and a stable climate (Carney, 2021).

These qualities are important to counter the negative aspects of knowl-edge-based leadership, including a focus on facts and figures rather than on people and the impact that decisions have on their lives. The danger of an over emphasis on knowledge-based decisions is in the tendency to further research and examine the problem rather than focusing on solutions and taking swift action based upon risks, despite the uncertainty of the evidence. The benefits of utilising knowledge include informing strategic direction for effective solu-tions whilst monitoring progress and outcomes. During the pandemic, we saw how improving self-knowledge of reactions during emergencies and threats to life are keys to creating wise, calm, and compassionate responses that allow for clear and rapid decision-making.

Revisiting how evolution has influenced and shaped the expression of leadership, we can also consider the fundamental principles of how ecologi-cal and life systems can be applied to improve how leaders can effectively address our complex challenges. An ecological perspective enables us to see the whole picture with an appreciation that all life is inter-connected. Actions and the exchange of energy in one area affect other areas, often with rein-forcing feedback loops. Other key principles include ecological diversity and adaptability, which enables greater resilience across life systems (Nurse et al, 2010). The role of information and communication systems has recently been described as an ecological principle (O'Connor et al, 2019). Furthermore, combining ecological principles with a greater understanding of the applica-tion of complex adaptive systems has the potential to improve our responses to such complex situations as the poly-crisis (Fidanboy, 2022). As humanity cannot rely upon individual leaders to address the multiple threats to life, the last chapter applies these approaches in the form of a framework to strengthen Global Governance for People and Planet.

Key Messages

- **Transforming Leadership for Complexity and the Poly-crisis:** we need to actively train and develop leaders to address our multiple interacting global challenges including future pandemics and the planetary emergency.
- **Balancing the Art and Science of Leadership for Existential Threats:** the development of political leaders and policymakers requires a balanced mix of core scientific and art-based skills to respond effectively to our future threats to global and human security in order to interpret, plan, respond to, and communicate risks.
- **An Ecological Leadership Framework for Complex Global Challenges:** to enhance the ability to influence and shape dynamic and complex adaptive systems, whilst balancing evolutionary leadership skill sets of values and knowledge patterns whilst moderating dominance behaviours.
  - **Values – The Heart of Leadership:** establishing global ethical values for human and planetary responsibility can help navigate chaos and uncertainty with collaborative multi-lateral responses.
  - **Knowledge – Dynamic Skills for People and Planet:** the development of balanced multi-disciplinary skills and experience in dealing with emergencies, threats to humanity, risks, preparedness, and responses.
  - **Dominance – Coordination and Governance for Emergency Leadership:** effective emergency responses benefit from command-and-control leadership to ensure security, combined with collaborative and coordinated action based upon a quiet ego whilst minimising the expression of negative power.

Bibliography

Adair J, (2002) '*Effective Strategic Leadership – An Essential Path to Success Guided by the World's Great Leaders*' Pan Macmillan.
Carney M, (2021) '*Value(s) – Building a Better World for All*' William Collins.
Cleary T, (1990) '*The Book of Leadership and Strategy – Lessons of the Chinese Masters*' Shambhala.
Desyatnikov R, (2020) 'Management in Crisis: the Best Leadership Style to Adopt in Times of Crisis' Forbes: https://www.forbes.com/sites/forbestechcouncil/2020/07/17/management-in-crisis-the-best-leadership-style-to-adopt-in-times-of-crisis/?sh=15f40d9e7cb4
Dror Y, (2017) '*For Rulers – Priming Political Leaders for Saving Humanity from Itself*' Westphalia Press.
Fidanboy M, (2022) '*Organisations and Complex Adaptive Systems*' Routledge.
Gardner D, (2009) 'Risk – the Science and Politics of Fear' Virgin Books.
Goleman D, (2002) '*The New Leaders – Transforming the Art of Leadership into the Science of Results*' Sphere.
Harari Y N, (2018) '*21 Lessons for the 21st Century*' Penguin.

HBR (2011) 'One Leadership' Harvard Business Review.

IAC (1997) 'Universal Declaration of Human Responsibilities' The InterAction Council: https://www.interactioncouncil.org/publications/universal-declaration-human-responsibilities

Kaufman S B et al, (2019) 'The Light vs Dark Triad of Personality: Contrasting Two Very Different Profiles of Human Nature' Frontiers of Psychology: https://www.frontiersin.org/articles/10.3389/fpsyg.2019.00467/full

Lowder T, (2007) 'New Dimensions of Leadership toward a Dynamic Model: A Synthesis of Transformational and Servant Leadership' Research Gate: https://www.researchgate.net/publication/228136394_New_Dimensions_of_Leadership_Toward_a_Dynamic_Model_A_Synthesis_of_Transformational_and_Servant_Leadership

Newton R et al, (2023) 'How to Become a Transformational Leader' London School of Economics: https://www.lse.ac.uk/study-at-lse/online-learning/insights/how-to-become-a-transformational-leader

Nurse J, Basher D, Bone A and Bird W, (2010) "An Ecological Approach to Promoting Population Mental Health and Well-being – A Response to the Challenge of Climate Change" *Perspectives in Public Health* 130(1): 27–33.

O'Connor M I et al, (2019) 'Principles of Ecology Revisited: Integrated Information and Ecological Theories for a More Unified Science' *Frontiers of Ecological Evolution* Vol 7: https://www.frontiersin.org/articles/10.3389/fevo.2019.00219/full

Rosling H et al, (2018) '*Factfulness-Ten Reasons we're Wrong about the World- and Why Things are Better than you Think*' Sceptre.

United Nations 'Leadership in Emergencies Toolkit' UN Emergency Preparedness and Support Team: accessed January 2023: https://hr.un.org/sites/hr.un.org/files/Leadership_in_Emergencies_Toolkit.pdf

Westen D, (2007) '*The Political Brain – the Role of Emotion in Deciding the Fate of Nations*' Public Affairs, Perseus Books Group.

Zohar D, (2021) '*Twelve Principles of Quantum Leadership*' Zero Distance, Palgrave, Macmillan, Singapore.

9 Future Proofing Global Security for People and Planet

Our Global Security System – Fit for the Future?

The world has failed to prevent the COVID-19 pandemic. And the next pandemic is just around the corner, whether it is from a new variant, avian influenza, or a genetically engineered pathogen. However, with exhausted health systems, struggling economies, competing conflicts, and multiple environmental catastrophes, we are even less resilient and prepared than we were at the beginning of the COVID-19 pandemic. Moreover, the pandemic revealed how unprepared our overall systems are for global shocks, with the majority of our world economy shutting down by 20% within the first part of 2020 (Tooze, 2021). However, our next pandemic could be a lot worse, for example, the avian influenza (H5NI) strain has a 50% mortality rate in the 870 humans that have contracted it in the last 20 years. With increasing spread between animals, it is potentially only a matter of time before the virus is able to transmit between humans (Tufekci, 2023). We desperately need to learn lessons from the COVID-19 pandemic, which should be seen as a gamechanger for leadership and how we strengthen governance mechanisms going forward (Ansell et al, 2020).

Significantly, a key learning from this pandemic was the absence of leaders that were able to advocate for an effective global strategic response. Although there were many heroic efforts by individual countries and leaders, these were insufficient on their own to change what became the predominant populist narrative. Although we need to enhance and transform the skills of individual leaders to respond effectively to emergencies and threats to human security going forward, on its own this will never be enough. In essence, we cannot rely upon the right leaders coming forward at the right time with the ability to influence and garner an effective multi-lateral response. Moreover, as pandemics spread with exponential speed, we need pre-existing systems in place that can be stood up and implemented rapidly. In order to ensure that our global security systems are fit for the purpose to prevent future pandemics requires the rapid application of learning from this pandemic. In particular, we need to establish fail-safe systems that can be triggered to prevent catastrophes

DOI: 10.1201/9781003181088-9

from occurring that do not rely upon individual failings. Moreover, as we sleep walk into our planetary emergency, we need to apply these lessons to address other threats to health, life, and existence. To achieve this requires building upon and fixing our existing governance infrastructure, which will be described in the following sections.

Existing Global Security Mechanisms for Health Threats:

The World Health Organization (WHO) is the designated United Nations lead Agency for Health, including health security, and is governed by the Executive Board and World Health Assembly (WHA), which consists of Health Ministers from member states. The WHO in turn reports to the United Nations General Assembly (UNGA) and General Committee, whereby member states can propose resolutions to the WHO WHA or UNGA, which express intent, however, these are generally not legally enforceable. The International Health Regulations (IHR) is one of the few legally binding instruments covering 196 countries that stipulate responsibilities for countries to report the emergence of public health events and epidemics that constitute a 'Public Health Emergency of International Concern' (PHEIC).

Whilst the Global Preparedness Monitoring Board and the Independent Panel for Pandemic Preparedness and Response produce annual reports for the WHA outlining risks and making recommendations, they are not enforceable. A review of the current (2005) IHR is under way due to the failure of the effectiveness of response to the COVID-19 pandemic. Moreover, at the initiative of the European Union and other Member States, the WHO is coordinating the development of a stronger legal requirement in the form of a Pandemic Treaty. However, in its current form, it is unclear how the Treaty will interact with the IHR. Moreover, the draft Pandemic Treaty as it stands is unlikely to be sufficient in preventing future pandemics. This is in part due to a lack of overall investment, combined with disincentives to reporting and the hazards inherent in a Treaty that relies upon member states taking individual responsibility.

There are a number of other International and United Nations organisations that contribute to health emergencies, such as the World Bank, UNICEF, the United Nations Office for the Coordination of Humanitarian Affairs (OCHA), the UN Disaster Assessment and Coordination (UNDAC), and the Sendai Framework for Disaster Risk Reduction. However, they also have their own funding and competing mandates and variably cooperate with the WHO and wider health sector. Although there are a multitude of philanthropists and donors, such as the Wellcome Trust and the Bill and Melinda Gates Foundation, GAVI, and more recently COVAX and the ACT Accelerator, that contribute to pandemic response, many are motivated by their own agendas and overly influenced by pharmaceutical companies. For example, the majority of donor funding has focused upon medical interventions, treatment, and research. In contrast, minimal investment has gone into strengthening public health services and capacity as part of the health system, which forms the foundation of prevention.

Prior to the pandemic, the Global Outbreak and Response Network (GOARN) was already in operation and consists of a network of partners, laboratories, and institutions coordinated by the WHO to investigate infectious disease risks that pose an epidemic threat. Whilst following the pandemic, a number of G7 countries have established partnerships with the WHO, for a range of pandemic centres. However, these centres, along with organisations such as the Global Health Security Agenda, are largely driven by high-income countries and are seen by low-and middle-income countries as motivated primarily to protect rich populations and interests. Many of these bodies have different and independent agendas that are not fully accountable to the WHO, representative of all member states, or the United Nations governance architecture. The multitude of COVID-19 digital apps created in the pandemic, with approximately 100 countries producing their own version, can be seen as symbolic of the repetition of efforts and the relative lack of global strategic coordination that occurred throughout the pandemic (P4PPPa, 2022).

A Global Security Framework for People and Planet

At first glance, the multitude of existing partners and global security mechanisms for health threats appears to be comprehensive, and in many respects, it can be seen that there are a wealth of initiatives addressing the different aspects of health security. However, a key challenge has been the ability of the WHO to coordinate these many initiatives with the authority and ability to influence heads of government and financing mechanisms. Moreover, as health is seen as an expert field, the majority of responses involve health bodies interacting with others across the health sector. In essence, global health security, which is a relatively new concept in itself, operates within a bubble, in relative isolation from the mainstream resilience and security architecture. This means that when a crisis like the pandemic occurs, the mainstream security governance mechanisms often are slow to be applied to health threats. In many respects, a similar process has occurred with the environment and climate change which has largely been led by experts in these consecutive fields. However, going forward what is required is that threats to health and our planetary crisis need to be incorporated into our existing global security infrastructure (IAC, 2022).

The United Nations Security Council (UNSC) represents such a mechanism and is responsible for International Peace and Security, reporting to the UN General Assembly every year. The UN Security Council has powers to establish peacekeeping initiatives, international sanctions, binding resolutions, and military action. However, the Security Council mainly focuses upon military conflicts, and although, the Council passed a resolution presented by the USA on HIV/AIDs, the UK was unsuccessfully in proposing a resolution on climate change and global security. This highlights a significant gap in the international architecture of a high-level multi-lateral mechanism to coordinate and respond to non-military global security challenges such as pandemics and the climate emergency. Furthermore, the Security Council consists of five permanent members, including China, France, Russia, the UK, and the USA, any of which have the power to veto any substantive resolution, which has compromised its ability to be fully effective.

The conflict driven by Russia combined with the pandemic and the increasing threats from our planetary emergency illustrates the increasing need to modernise our global security infrastructure in order to address the full range of existential threats that we now face today and into the future. Drawing upon existing strengths whilst addressing gaps and weaknesses in our current global security infrastructure we have the opportunity to prevent future pandemics and apply learning for the planetary emergency. Reporting to the UNGA with links to the UN Security Council, the creation of a Global Security Council for People and Planet is proposed (IAC, 2022). This could include strengthening governance and political leadership for prevention, risk reduction, and emergency responses for people and planet. The council could enhance capacity and coordinate responses from across the main components illustrated in the 'Global Security Framework for Planet and People' below, and instigate collaborative solutions to address relative gaps (Figure 9.1).

Securing adequate and long-term investment for global health security has always been a challenge, as it has largely been seen as a voluntary sector, based upon charitable funding. In contrast, military security has rarely struggled for funding. Going forward will require new funding mechanisms that do not distort the WHO's remit and reframe the importance of collective insurance

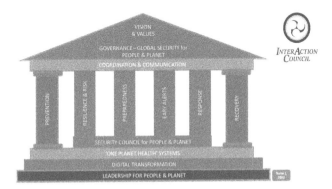

Figure 9.1 A Global Security Framework for People and Planet

against threats from global risks (Brown, 2021). Financial mechanisms need to be adopted that encourage sustainable investment in global goods such as the health of humans, as well as the environment and ensuring we have a liveable planet. However, the proposed council could draw upon the multitude of existing resources and initiatives, further enhancing these with an adaptable strategic framework, ranging from Prevention to Recovery. This could engage multiple partners to create an integrated multi-sector systems response with a strong focus on prevention and risk reduction from our complex and multiple security challenges. Furthermore, the council could play a key role in transforming leadership and developing capacity to strengthen governance mechanisms that prevent and respond to emergencies with the goal of securing the well-being of future generations (IAC, 2022).

The council could be supported by a Digital Platform with a small team to act as a Secretariat that enhances collaborative action, coordination, and communication of existing organisations. The platform could deliver at speed and scale by the application of digital technology (P4PPP, 2022). Such a council and platform could provide an on-going international infrastructure that convenes on a regular basis to assess global human, animal, and planetary risks to human health, life, and existence, including the risks of planetary tipping points. The platform and council could play a key role in communicating early alerts to political leaders, and garnering multi-lateral resources and responses to intervene early, contain dangers, and reduce harm. Membership of the council could be drawn from Regional and World Leaders and Heads of Government that represent our diverse populations from around the world. Whilst the platform could combine the wider perspectives of multi-sector experts and decision-makers, in order to identify appropriate levels of responses to risks. Existing digital tools could be applied to enhance the speed and reach of modern 'One Planet Health' Systems with an integrated multi-sector workforce, including strengthening leadership for people and planet (P4PPP, 2022).

Threats to Health, Life, and Existence – An Integrated Global Security Response

There is an increasing recognition by senior world leaders of the need to take a strategic approach to addressing existential threats from pandemics and our planetary emergency as well as nuclear war and conflicts (The Elders, 2023). Furthermore, the United Nations Secretary General is leading an initiative called 'Our Common Agenda', which builds upon a series of engagement exercises and a Foresight report (UN, 2023), that has prioritised five elements to potentially advance, including:

- A UN Futures Lab
- A UN Summit on the Future in 2024
- A UN Envoy for Future Generations

- Periodic UN Strategic Foresight and Global Threats Report
- A Repurposed UN Trustee Council as a Multi-Stakeholder Foresight Body

The Foresight report outlines a range of potential elements and actions to take forward with Member States and Civil Society Partners, including the concept of an UN Office of Existential Threats reporting to the UN Secretary General. This represents an important shift in our International Family coming together to address risks for our global security. However, going forward, such initiatives will only be successful if they can do more than describe the problems. This will require recognising the interconnected aspects of our multiple and complex challenges, described as a 'poly-crisis' in order to identify successful strategic pathways through our existential crisis. Strengthening and modernising global governance for dealing with these interconnected threats, including pandemics, the planetary emergency, and conflicts will be crucial going forward.

Embedding multiple security risks under an umbrella mechanism within the UN system could act to transform how we address our multiple existential threats. Such an integrated council could coordinate and engage Member States, Civil Society, and Young Leaders with a Declaration for the Future. As with the pandemic, a greater emphasis on preventing and reducing risks is required combined with early warning systems that trigger rapid interventions. Furthermore, sharing knowledge to inform and scale scientific and technological advances need to be combined with nature-based solutions. The World Academy of Art and Science is advancing such an integrated approach to addressing existential threats that focus upon system enabler solutions including governance, knowledge, advocacy, and capacity building and is illustrated below (Nurse, 2023). Securing our future will be dependent upon building capacity for wise and courageous leaders which is described in the following section (Figure 9.2).

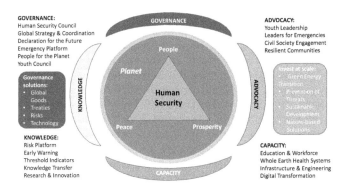

Figure 9.2 A Governance Framework for Existential Threats to Human Security

Cultivate Wise and Courageous Leaders to Secure our Future

Going forward, we can conclude that the world needs to cultivate balanced wise and courageous leaders to be able to navigate humanity's way through multiple complex challenges, chaos, and uncertainty, in order to create a liveable world for all to share. The components of wise leadership can be described as perception, authenticity, patience, and courage (Stebbins, 2022). In the context of pandemics and our planetary emergency, perception can be seen as the ability to see the whole picture from a global perspective. This involves being adaptable, intuitive, and open to what is not known, with the ability to engage others and create balanced decisions. Whilst authenticity is about self-awareness, honesty, integrity, and being values driven, with the ability to learn from mistakes. Patience involves the ability to manage negative emotions and behaviours in one-self and others and requires humility, resilience, and a quiet ego in order to remain calm and make sound and sustainable judgements.

In contrast, courage provides heart-centred leadership, with a strong vision of creating a better world, whilst enabling others to navigate calamity with compassion. To become a wise leader requires learning from experience, cultivating personal virtues including humility, self-restraint, magnanimity, commitment, and courage (McKenna and Rooney, 2019). This requires the ability to balance our ancestorial drivers of leadership, by emphasising positive values as a basis to restrain the desire for dominance, personal power, wealth, and other negative traits. These qualities combine with experience, knowledge, and skills to successfully navigate emergencies, complexity, and conflicts.

To achieve this will require a change in culture and that these attributes are actively selected for and developed in those that stand for political and policy leadership roles (Hardman, 2022). For example, we saw how several low-ego style and female leaders were successfully able to navigate the pandemic by emphasising values that placed people first. This enabled swift decisions to be made during chaos and uncertainty, which resulted in less harm to both health and to the economy. Going forward, to create wise, resilient and balanced leadership will require actively drawing our future leaders from across all our communities in order to represent all aspects of our diverse world. To achieve this will require proactive training, values-based motivation, mentoring, and selection processes to cultivate our future leaders, especially from under-represented and disempowered groups, both within our societies and from around the world (Gillard and Okonjo-Iweala, 2020). This can be reinforced by the creation of fair, diverse, and inclusive cultures that emphasise social and emotional intelligence, collaboration, and responsibility towards others. Whilst applying effective interventions that address bullying and antisocial childhood behaviour disorders has the potential to reduce the occurrence of negative leadership patterns that emerge as adult psychopathic behaviours (Bellis et al, 2017).

The establishment of the UN and multi-lateral agencies following the World Wars marked a significant shift in global governance for security and cooperation. However, our global security infrastructure was designed for the last century's challenges and requires substantial reform and renewal to become fit for purpose for the challenges in this century. Furthermore, learning from the successes of former world leaders has the potential to guide us through our future challenges. For example, the experience of navigating intransigent conflicts to reach a compromise built upon fairness was key to HE Bertie Aherns role in bringing together partners for the Irish 'Good Friday Agreement'. Furthermore, the foundational principles of fairness and compromise will need to be at the heart of achieving a successful resolution for a Brexit agreement in Northern Ireland (O'Carroll, 2023). The wisdom, vision, advocacy, and soft diplomacy skills of former political leaders who are committed to working together, often behind the scenes have been critical in creating a safer world for all. Groups of former national and world leaders such as the InterAction Council, the Club of Rome, the Club of Madrid, and the Elders have been instrumental in overcoming conflict and bringing about peace, whilst raising the political agenda in response to our planetary crisis.

The exceptional ability of a handful of leaders, such as Mahatma Gandhi and Nelson Mandela, has transformed the injustices of colonial oppression through the values of reconciliation and non-violence. Whilst African leaders such as President Olusegun Obasanjo from Nigeria were instrumental in supported the creation of the African Union, other leaders have helped maintain and forge peace between their neighbours, including Oscar Arias Sanchez Nobel Peace Prize laureate from Costa Rica, and Abdel Salam Majali former Prime minister of Jordan. The political insight, networks, and gravitas afforded by those who have been national as well as world leaders, including Helen Clark and Gro Harlem Brundtland, have proved invaluable in providing future direction to prevent further pandemics. Going forward, advancing intergenerational leadership initiatives such as the InterAction Council partnership with One Young World (OYW, 2023) has the potential to fast-track leadership skills by harnessing the wisdom of former leaders, in combination with the energy and passion of young leaders.

Ensuring that we cultivate the sort of leaders that we need to address our current and future challenges whilst securing a sustainable world for all will become increasingly essential. Moreover, to be successful in saving the world from catastrophe will require leaders coming forth that combine wisdom and courageousness along with collaborative and diplomatic skills driven by a sense of urgency. Rather than continuing with our default approach of letting the most dominant and power-oriented leaders emerge, will require the active cultivation of leaders across the life course. This will involve transforming our education systems to develop multi-disciplinary knowledge reorientated to the skillsets required for creating a sustainable world, such as the Commonwealth Curriculum that enables lifelong learning for delivering the Sustainable Development Goals (Commonwealth, 2017). The application of existing educational systems combined with Massive Open Online Learning (MOOCS) has the potential to scale up and modernise quality education around the world.

Furthermore, aligning education with workforce planning to secure our futures will require embedding skills within examination syllabuses and professional development programmes. Such a workforce needs to operate within a coordinated local to global system, consisting of a balanced mix of community practitioners, emergency and operational workers, experts, professionals, and policymakers as well as drawing upon wider allied workforces. Identifying common values and principles, such as those held by Rotary and other international alliances, has the potential to unify and reinforce efforts across a diverse local to global multi-professional workforce. In particular, the transformation of education and training programmes for public health and environmental health professionals and practitioners has the potential to develop into a dynamic transdisciplinary 'One Planet Health Systems' workforce. This could include developing leaders from existing Public Health, Environmental Health, Earth Systems, Global Health, Planetary Health, and One Health backgrounds, which are capable of protecting and promoting the health of humans, animals, the environment, and the planet in order to secure the well-being of our future generations.

Recommendations – Towards a Safe, Fair, Healthy, and Sustainable World for All

In summary, we stand at a pivotal moment in human civilisation, whereby we have the potential to apply learning from past catastrophes to transform the trajectory of human health, life, and existence. Even within an Emergency Room (ER) situation, there is always hope to revive a moribund patient, who is later able to recover and flourish. However, in order to secure our future existence will require the transformation of our leaders and our leadership systems. This will depend upon the ability of wise and courageous leaders enabled by ethical principles with robust global security governance structures. The recommendations below build upon learning from the COVID-19 pandemic, and outline the key components required to address our global threats to health, life, and existence and create a safe, fair, healthy, and sustainable world for all.

Recommendations

1 **Global Ethical Principles for People and Planet:** for collaborative action to address existential threats, with equity and the protection of global

goods including health, oceans, and the environment to secure the well-being of future generations; emphasise political responsibilities to support multi-lateral responses, and to enhance trust and rapid decision-making where uncertainty exists in addressing challenges during pandemics and the climate crisis.

2 **A Global Security Council for People and Planet:** to facilitate multi-lateral leadership with heads of government with an emphasis on preventing emergencies, and enabling coordinated and strategic responses; maintains oversight of emerging and early risks, triggering rapid action through the UN, countries, and partner organisations to intervene early to risks and evolving emergencies, garnering political support, resources, and multi-lateral leadership.

3 **A Platform on Global Security for People and Planet:** utilising digital technology to coordinate existing infrastructure and initiatives for integrated risk assessments and early warning systems linked to adaptable multi-sector Prevention, Preparedness, and Emergency Responses; build upon existing frameworks, tools, organisations, partnerships, and resources; enhance legislation, policies, financing and accountability mechanisms including independent Quality Assurance, to strengthen and modernise governance systems at all levels; where gaps exist, co-create tools to enable governance mechanisms and systems strengthening.

4 **Insure and Invest in a Healthy Planet for All:** around the world, invest a minimum of US $2 per person per year for pandemic prevention, preparedness, and response; reframe the Environment and Health as Global Goods requiring investment and insurance in order to prevent future pandemics and the planetary emergency; and prioritise investments to create a rapid transition to net zero, combined with recovering earth systems that have a high risk of tipping points for escalating the climate crisis, including oceans and water, air, land, and food systems, with Scientific and Nature-Based Solutions.

5 **Create One Planet Health Systems:** to strengthen security, resilience, and sustainable well-being at community, country, and global levels; building upon and modernising existing operations, services, resources, and organisations; and to create and enable robust multi-sector systems with enhanced coordination, infrastructure, leadership, and workforce capacity. Draw upon and modernise existing professions and initiatives including Environmental Health, Public Health, Planetary Health, and One Health to strengthen health systems for humans, animals, and the planet.

6 **Emergency Leadership skills and capacity at all levels and backgrounds:** to prevent, interpret risks, prepare for, respond to, and recovery from, emergencies as part of an all-hazards approach to address all threats to life and existence, with an enhanced focus on pandemics and the planetary emergency; supported by enhancing scientific and risk literacy, with skills for collaborative working and communications, combined with the application of ethical principles for decision-making, priority setting,

strategy development and delivery, enabled by robust governance mechanisms with transparent processes.

7   **Cultivate Wise and Courageous Leaders – A Workforce for the Future:** learn from successful leaders on applying transformational and dynamic leadership styles; future transdisciplinary and diverse leadership needs to be cultivated through education, training, professional development, and leadership programmes, to promote a 'One Planet Health Systems' workforce. Align education, skills, professional and workforce development, and resources to respond to emergencies and existential threats to secure a healthy planet for a prosperous and peaceful future for all.

8   **Scale Collaborative Action through Digital Transformation:** to enhance risk management and governance with rapid responses and accessible communications to multi-sector audiences; empower communities and countries with open access, reliable information, and digital tools; ensure digital governance to prevent misinformation, hacking, and scams; enhance efficient ways of working, with reduced travel, and the creation of efficient and green digital systems; strengthen leadership and workforce capacity supported with online learning, networks and forums; connect, share learning, enable collaborative partnerships and promote research and innovative solutions on Global Security Challenges for Planet and People.

Bibliography

Ansell C, Sørensen E and Torfing J, (2020) 'The COVID-19 Pandemic as a Game Changer for Public Administration and Leadership? The Need for Robust Governance Responses to Turbulent Problems' *Public Management Review*, https://doi.org/ 10.1080/14719037.2020.1820272: https://doi.org/10.1080/14719037.2020.1820272

Bellis M A, Hardcastle K, Hughes K, Wood S and Nurse J, (2017): 'Preventing Violence, Promoting Peace: A Policy Toolkit for Preventing Interpersonal, Collective and Extremist Violence' Public Health Wales and the Commonwealth Secretariat: https://phwwhocc.co.uk/resources/preventing-violence-promoting-peace-a-policy-toolkit-for-preventing-interpersonal-collective-and-extremist-violence/

Brown G, (2021) '*Seven Ways to Change the World – How to Fix the Most Pressing Problems we Face*' Simon and Schuster.

Commonwealth (2017) 'Curriculum Framework for Enabling the Sustainable Development Goals' The Commonwealth Secretariat, London, UK: https://www.thecommonwealth-ilibrary.org/index.php/comsec/catalog/book/1064

Gillard J and Okonjo-Iweala N, (2020) '*Women and Leadership – Real Lives, Real Lessons*' Penguin.

Hardman I, (2022) '*Why We Get the Wrong Politicians*' Atlantic Books.

IAC (2022) 'Ending the Pandemic - Enhancing Global Security for Planet and People, A Framework for the Future' The InterAction Council: https://www.interactioncouncil. org/sites/default/files/Pandemic%20Exit%20Strategy%20reduced.pdf

McKenna B and Rooney D, (2019) 'Wise Leadership' Chapter 29, Part VII: Wisdom in Action; Sternberg RJ and Gluck J (Eds) '*The Cambridge Handbook of Wisdom*' ();Cambridge University Press.

Nurse J, (2023) '*Human Security and Existential Threats – A Governance Framework for Planet, Peace, People and Prosperity*' Cadmus, World Academy of Art and Science.

O'Carroll L, (2023) 'Solving Northern Ireland Brexit Dispute not Rocket Science Bertie Ahern Says' https://www.theguardian.com/uk-news/2023/jan/23/solving-northern-ireland-brexit-dispute-not-rocket-science-bertie-ahern-says

OYW (2023) 'One Young World x InterAction Council: Exclusive Mentorship Sessions' One Young World: https://www.oneyoungworld.com/blog/one-young-world-x-interaction-council-exclusive-mentorship-sessions

P4PPP (2022a) 'Creating Digital Solutions for Pandemics and Global Health Security' Platform for Planet Place and People, The Commonwealth Centre for Digital Health: https://sites.google.com/view/p4ppp/resources

P4PPP (2022b) 'Creating Digital Futures: Platform for Planet, Place and People, (P4PPP); Progress and Plans 2022-2027' https://sites.google.com/view/p4ppp/resources

P4PPP (2023) 'Digital Solutions for our Planetary Emergency – Creating Common Goods for Global Security' Platform for Planet Place and People (P4PPP); TBP.

Rotary International (2023) https://www.rotary.org/en/our-causes

Stebbins G, (2022) 'The Four Foundations of Wise Leaders' Forbes: https://www.forbes.com/sites/forbescoachescouncil/2022/09/21/the-four-foundations-of-wise-leaders/?sh=5c92ab7569d0

The Elders (2023) 'The Elders – Working for Peace, Justice, Human Rights and a Sustainable Planet; Strategy 2023-2027': https://theelders.org/sites/default/files/newsarticaldocument/20230124-The-Elders-Strategy-2023-2027-for-web.pdf

Tooze A, (2021) '*Shutdown – How COVID Shook the World's Economy*' Viking.

Tufekci Z, (2023) 'An Even Deadlier Pandemic Could Soon be Here' Opinion, New York Times: https://www.nytimes.com/2023/02/03/opinion/bird-flu-h5n1-pandemic.html

UN (2023) 'Five UN Foresight Elements of our Common Agenda' The Millennium Project, Global Futures Studies and Research: https://www.millennium-project.org/five-un-foresight-elements-of-our-common-agenda/

Index

Note: *Italic* page numbers refer to figures.

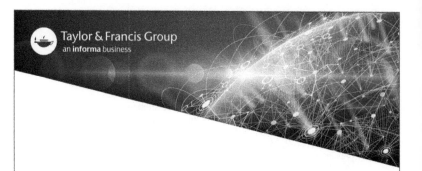

For Product Safety Concerns and Information please contact our EU
representative GPSR@taylorandfrancis.com
Taylor & Francis Verlag GmbH, Kaufingerstraße 24, 80331 München, Germany

www.ingramcontent.com/pod-product-compliance
Ingram Content Group UK Ltd.
Pitfield, Milton Keynes, MK11 3LW, UK
UKHW021057080625
459435UK00004B/38

* 9 7 8 1 0 3 2 0 1 0 0 3 8 *